3 2410 01839 9132

P9-DYD-423

MA

MAIN LIBRARY
PUBLIC LIBRARY
ST. PETERSBURG, FL

Your Brain After Chemo

Your Brain After Chemo

*A Practical Guide to Lifting the Fog
and Getting Back Your Focus*

DAN SILVERMAN, M.D., PH.D., AND IDELLE DAVIDSON

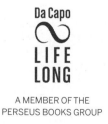

Da Capo
LIFE
LONG

A MEMBER OF THE
PERSEUS BOOKS GROUP

Many of the designations used by manufacturers and sellers to distinguish their products are claimed as trademarks. Where those designations appear in this book and Da Capo Press was aware of a trademark claim, the designations have been printed in initial capital letters.

Copyright © 2009 by Daniel Silverman and Idelle Davidson

All rights reserved. No part of this publication may be reproduced, stored in a retrieval system, or transmitted, in any form or by any means, electronic, mechanical, photocopying, recording, or otherwise, without the prior written permission of the publisher. Printed in the United States of America. For information, address Da Capo Press, 11 Cambridge Center, Cambridge, MA 02142.

Designed by Anita Koury
Set in 11.5 point Whitman by the Perseus Books Group

Library of Congress Cataloging-in-Publication Data
Silverman, Dan, 1956-
Your brain after chemo: a practical guide to lifting the fog and getting back your focus /
Dan Silverman and Idelle Davidson. —1st Da Capo Press ed.
        p. cm. .
    Includes bibliographical references and index.
    ISBN 978-0-7382-1259-3
1. Cancer—Chemotherapy—Complications. 2. Cognitive disorders. 3. Cancer—
Patients—Rehabilitation. I. Davidson, Idelle. II. Title.
RC271.C5S533 2009
616.99'4061—dc22

                          2009014030

Published by Da Capo Press
A Member of the Perseus Books Group
www.dacapopress.com

Note: The information in this book is true and complete to the best of our knowledge. This book is intended only as an informative guide for those wishing to know more about health issues. In no way is this book intended to replace, countermand, or conflict with the advice given to you by your own physician. The ultimate decision concerning care should be made between you and your doctor. We strongly recommend you follow his or her advice. Information in this book is general and is offered with no guarantees on the part of the authors or Da Capo Press. The authors and publisher disclaim all liability in connection with the use of this book. Some of the names in this book have been changed.

Da Capo Press books are available at special discounts for bulk purchases in the U.S. by corporations, institutions, and other organizations. For more information, please contact the Special Markets Department at the Perseus Books Group, 2300 Chestnut Street, Suite 200, Philadelphia, PA 19103, or call (800) 810–4145, ext. 5000, or e-mail special.markets@perseusbooks.com.

10 9 8 7 6 5 4 3 2 1

Contents

Foreword vii

Idelle's Story: Have We Met? ix

Part I: Talking With Your Oncologist

1   A Vulnerable Time 3

2   Rethinking "Chemo Brain" 8

3   Q & A With Your Doctor 13

Part II: Symptoms and Signs

4   I Found My Keys, But I Lost Myself 31

5   Relationships 38

6   Multitasking, Word Retrieval, Memory,
    and Concentration 44

7   Fatigue and Depression 55

8   Measuring Forgetfulness 61

9   Body of Evidence 71

Part III: Molecules Behaving Badly

10   The Healthy Brain 79

11   The Unhealthy Brain 86

12   Hormones—His and Hers 99

Part IV: Getting Your Brain Back on Track

13 Depressing Days? 121

14 Sleeping Through Insomnia 134

15 Fatigue, Inattention, and Poor Concentration 143

16 Fear, Stress, and Mindfulness 156

17 Brain Food 172

18 Some Tips for (Re)Organizing Your
    Day-to-Day Life 191

Part V: How to Reclaim Your Brain Chemistry

19 Nine Daily Steps You Can Start Doing Today 201

20 Summary of the Nine Steps and Worksheet 221

21 Future Directions 225

Authors' Notes 239

Acknowledgments 241

Resources 247

Generic Drugs and Brand Name Equivalents 255

Notes 257

Index 273

Foreword

Perhaps you picked up this book because you recently were diagnosed with cancer, or with a new stage of cancer, and you and your doctors are contemplating various chemotherapy regimens as part of your upcoming therapy. If so, this book will provide state-of-the art-knowledge to empower you to be as informed as possible when making decisions that may affect the well-being of your body and mind for a very long time to come.

Perhaps you've already had cancer and chemotherapy, and you find it's taking all your concentration just to make it through this paragraph, something that never would have happened prior to chemo. On the other hand, perhaps making it this far has not been particularly difficult, but you're still not mentally functioning at the high level you were before chemotherapy. In either case, if you're eager to learn what can be done to get your brain working better faster, you've come to the right place.

Why this particular book? Idelle's experiences both as a medical journalist as well as a cancer (and chemo) survivor (she'll tell you more about this in the next section) are ideally suited for articulating the challenges that she and hundreds of other patients with whom she has communicated have faced and, in many cases, overcome.

Also, this book conveys what I have discovered as a doctor who has seen thousands of patients with cancer and neurological problems, as well as a physician-scientist who for many years has been conducting research that's aimed at decreasing chemotherapy- related problems. Within that work, my colleagues and I continue to capture images that reveal areas of diminished metabolism in the brain tissue of patients who suffer from cognitive difficulties as much as five to ten years after their last dose of chemotherapy. These brain abnormalities correspond to their decreased ability to get through the words on a page, accurately recall paragraphs or pictures they looked at thirty minutes earlier, or even to simply feel clear-minded. In other words, we can literally see and measure in these brain images biological changes that our patients experience as "chemo brain" or "chemo fog."

Finally, this book is not just a source of the best biomedical information available on the subject, but it is also a straightforward and evidence-based "how-to" manual for people facing the prospect or the reality of a decline in thinking abilities after cancer and chemotherapy. In essence, it has been written to help people reclaim not only the health of their bodies, but also the whole of who they really are.

—*Dan Silverman, M.D., Ph.D.*

Idelle's Story
Have We Met?

I'm a little like Groucho Marx: He didn't wish to belong to any club that would accept someone like him as a member. But one club won't take my "no" for an answer. So here is what I tell it: *"Do not call. Do not even whisper my name. GET ME THE HELL OUT!"*

If you are reading this, then you or someone you care about may have been invited into this club, too. I never asked to join. None of us does. The post office clearly got the address wrong. I exercised. I ate organic foods. Heck, I'm a health writer! In fact, for three years I served as contributing editor to a cancer magazine. How's that for irony?

But somehow, the dark force that controls these things dragged me into the club in July 2005, as I kicked and screamed, wanting to tear its eyes out. That's when my gynecologist felt a lump in my right breast during a routine physical exam. A subsequent mammogram, ultrasound, MRI, and needle biopsy confirmed the worst: cancer.

My tumor was small. I opted for a lumpectomy. The bad news: Although the cancer had not metastasized and was still in its early stages, it had spread to two lymph nodes under my arm. That, said my surgeon Nova Foster—a woman to whom I am indebted for life for her skill and compassion—would earn me six rounds of chemotherapy and seven weeks of radiation treatments. It also earned me my experience with "chemo brain."

And still, there was more. I was among about 20 percent of women whose cancer cells make too much of a protein called HER-2. These tumors are particularly aggressive and are more likely to recur than other types of breast cancers.

But a breakthrough treatment that would dramatically improve my odds awaited me at UCLA's Jonsson Comprehensive Cancer Center. I happened to live just a few miles from the medical center. That was a plus. I also knew that UCLA was one of several comprehensive cancer sites that was studying a promising new drug called trastuzumab or its trade name, Herceptin, for early stage breast cancer. In fact, Dennis Slamon, the scientist who helped develop Herceptin, practiced at UCLA. My oncologist at the time worked with Dr. Slamon and served as principal investigator for the UCLA arm of the international study. Thankfully, she recommended me for the drug.

Herceptin is not chemotherapy. It is a monoclonal antibody that specifically targets cancer cells that over-express HER-2. Results from the trials published in the October 20, 2005, *New England Journal of Medicine* showed that patients with early stage breast cancer who received Herceptin in combination with chemotherapy cut their recurrence rate by half, compared to patients who received chemotherapy alone.

So in August 2005, more than a year before the Food and Drug Administration expanded the use of Herceptin to treat the general public for early stage HER-2 breast cancer (the FDA had already approved the antibody for metastatic or advanced breast cancer in 1998), I began twelve months of Herceptin treatments in combination with four-and-a-half months of standard chemotherapy.

I have read the club bylaws, and I've learned the secret handshake. There are benefits of membership. I am alive. That's a biggy. I will be forever grateful to my UCLA doctors, nurses, therapists, and technicians, those selfless individuals who shepherded me through the most difficult time of my life.

Then there is the other benefit—the awareness that cancer doesn't define you. It defines your friends and family. Some disappointed me: One long-time friend stopped calling after learning of my diagnosis.

But they were the exceptions. If nothing else, cancer illuminated the many angels in my life, those who stood oak-solid, no matter what. My husband, Peter, tops the list. I can't even count the nights during those months of treatment when I fell asleep sobbing in his arms, the fear so large in my chest that I could hardly breathe. I'd wake in the morning, his cheek against mine, his arms still around me, holding me safe.

For me, there was always the trust issue—who to tell, and who not. That may seem surprising, considering all the inspiring men, women, and children I have interviewed over the years who spoke candidly about their own cancer experiences. Former First Lady Betty Ford was one. When I met with her in 2001, in her home near Palm Springs, California, she was then eighty-three and as lovely and active as ever. She had soft, blue eyes and short hair that she wore brushed back from her intelligent face. Mostly, I remember her manner in that cheerful living room that was decorated in yellows and greens. "They're cool colors because it's hot in the desert," she said. She patted my hand. "Now tell me about yourself. . . . "

I understood how she might have charmed the pants off the media back in 1974. That was the year she went public with her own diagnosis and mastectomy. Until then, the "C" word was not discussed in polite company. Many women owe Betty Ford a debt of gratitude. She opened the floodgates for advocacy. She helped save countless lives.

Then there was Olympic gold medal ice skating champion Peggy Fleming who haltingly recalled the loss of her mother to multiple myeloma, a cancer of the bone marrow. She then told of her own struggle with breast cancer. And Queen Noor of Jordan, in her forested home near Washington, DC, overlooking the Potomac, sat with me on her sofa and described how she ached for her husband, King Hussein. He had died the year before of non-Hodgkin's B-cell lymphoma. "I will mourn all my life," she said.

There's a certain amount of detachment involved when you're a journalist, looking in. You write in the third person; you are the observer. But now *this* story was about the I, the me, the first person. That meant vulnerability. My friends and family offered to sit with me during my four-hour chemo infusions, but I turned most of them down flat. Call it denial—or pride—but I couldn't stand the idea of letting them see me as a cancer patient. I didn't want to subject them to hospital smells and patients with chest catheters and bald heads. Because forever after, that might be me in their mind's eye.

But I am human, after all. I learned that lesson when I started radiation treatments. I showed up alone, of course. One of the staff had assigned me the 9 a.m. appointments. I arrived promptly. This would be the first of thirty-seven almost-daily treatments. I followed the instructions given to me the week before: I stopped in the dressing room, changed into a gown, and stowed my belongings in a locker. I sat in the waiting room. It was now about ten minutes past nine o'clock. Within moments the technician called my name, and I followed her into the radiation bay.

There was no hello and welcome or thank you for choosing our airline, I will be your flight attendant. Instead, hand on her hip, she scolded me! Apparently I was to have arrived fifteen minutes prior to my appointment so that I could change and be ready at 9 a.m. sharp. I must *never* keep the technicians waiting past my appointment time, she said. They operate on a tight schedule, and I must never, ever, do that again!

I felt like a kindergartner on the first day of school, and my new teacher didn't like me. Tears stung my eyes. I followed her into an ice-cold room where I was told to uncover my right breast and lie on a table. She and an aide positioned my body so that it lined up precisely under the path of the X-ray beam. They did this quickly and clinically, cold hands on my breast, manipulating me this way and that.

Above me a humongous machine, hanging like a giant space alien on the ceiling, stared down at me. "We're going to leave the room now," she said. "But we'll be watching from a monitor just outside. You must remain still. No deep breaths. Don't move. Do not move!"

The machine, as if disembodied, creaked and angled itself to shoot its beams into me. I don't know if it was the scolding or the frightening arm of the machine like a tentacle, or that I was saturated with an emotional and physical weariness that I could no longer contain, but the tears rolled down my cheeks, and then came the sobs. Have you ever experienced uncontrollable weeping while remaining stock still? It's impossible. I could see my chest rising, and I heard the technician's voice blast from the intercom, "You need to stop crying. Stop crying now! Do we need to stop the machine?" I formed the word "no" and willed my mind to think of nothing.

But afterward, after I dressed and was walking back to my car, I pulled out my cell phone and called my husband at work. I couldn't reach him. Damn it, where the hell was he? I was furious. I needed him here with me, *now*. But I hadn't asked him to accompany me, and following my lead, he hadn't offered. I tried calling my sister, Carole, and brother, Charles. Usually we talk a couple of times during the day. No luck. My kids were not around, so that was no good. Then I called my cousin, Jan. She picked up right away, and I found myself crying so hard that I couldn't get the words out. All she heard was, "Late . . . cold . . . machine . . . terrifying . . . so scared."

I realized then that I could no longer pretend. I was needy after all—I was in need. I would never let anyone I love handle this alone. You bet I'd be there. And now I needed them here with me. It was then I joined a cancer support group and started asking my family and friends for help.

I discussed those days with my friend and cousin Marcia, a psychotherapist. She was ten years old when her mother died of ovarian cancer. She wasn't allowed in the hospital to see her mom. No one told her what was going on. She never said goodbye. "It would have been cathartic for me to go with you to treatment," she said. "I would have given to you what I was never permitted to give my mom." I wish I had known. We would have helped each other.

A few months later I attended a weeklong health retreat, complete with classes in meditation, nutrition, and spirituality. I was struck by the seminar leaders' use of language. In every instance, in place of the word "cancer," they used the words "health opportunity." How's that for spin? Yet I've come to believe that what I've gone through has connected me more deeply to those I love.

Except for the worst days when radiation treatment knocked the stuffing out of me, I kept writing and accepting freelance magazine assignments. I had finished chemo, but I still got Herceptin infusions every three weeks. During my good days, I'd throw on my wig and drive to Cedars-Sinai Medical Center in Los Angeles where I interviewed notable scientists about their breakthroughs. Those stories appeared in the Cedars-Sinai magazine, *Discoveries*. Some of the doctors I interviewed worked in cancer research. I'd meet with them and wonder, can they tell I'm in the "club"? Is my wig on straight?

For me, losing my hair because of chemotherapy wasn't that traumatic. I had interviewed enough cancer patients to expect it. What terrified me then was sitting in that communal chemo room and watching the drugs flow through my vein like Drano. I tried to imagine the chemo as "good guys," little Pac-men gobbling up all the evil cancer cells. But what was the chemo doing to my healthy cells?

I grew forgetful. As my friends in the cancer support group assured me, this was completely normal. Normal? Are you kidding? They'd exchange glances, chuckle, and tell me I had chemo brain just like the rest of them. Indeed, their stories were hilarious in a member-of-the-club kind of way. One told of running in and out of her home six times, first forgetting her purse, then her grocery list, then other items. Finally, totally flustered, she made it to the car only to realize she had locked her keys in the house!

My friend Joyce, also a psychotherapist, is undergoing treatment for ovarian cancer. One day when we were having lunch, Joyce confided she had written out a check and placed it in an envelope, planning to mail it later. When she went to seal the envelope, she noticed two checks inside to the same person. She had written a duplicate, one after the other, and hadn't noticed.

My first experience with chemo brain happened midway through chemotherapy. I was shopping at the Century City mall, a few miles from UCLA. It was almost dark, and I needed to get home.

I realized I had no idea where I parked my car. I had no clue which level I had parked on, which escalator I had used, or even which store appeared first as I entered the mall. I was mortified and too embarrassed to ask a security guard for help. I did find my car eventually but only after riding up and down every escalator in the mall, and only after setting off the car alarm button on my key chain. I imagine this is how people with Alzheimer's disease must feel when they become disoriented. My heart goes out to them.

Other incidents were less dramatic. I'd forget my sister's phone number or completely tune out when someone spoke to me. My college-aged sons, Ben and Matt, liked to tease me when it happened. "Oh Mom, don't worry about it," they'd say. "You've always had chemo brain!" Although I would laugh right along with those not-so-little monsters, believe me, I knew the difference.

I was concerned enough about my memory to discuss it with my current oncologist. He was not unsympathetic, but he suggested my problem might be more related to anxiety. And I have to admit, I do feel anxious each time I visit him. My reaction is not unlike that of a rabbi I know who had colon cancer and had experienced severe nausea from chemotherapy. Now years later, the moment he steps inside the lobby of his oncologist's office, he starts to gag.

My response is different but Pavlovian just the same. I associate my doctor with potentially bearing bad news. When I see him, I make sure my sneakers are double-knotted, so that the other shoe never drops. And although he's not a particularly touchy-feely kind of guy, he is kindhearted enough to reassure me each time we meet.

So yes, there's anxiety, but it lifts when I leave his office. My problems with memory and concentration remained for several months. But I think the mist has cleared or that I've learned tools to stay focused. There are ways to compensate, as you'll see.

You'll also see that there's plenty of science behind chemo brain, although some oncologists will tell you that this *idea* of mental fog is just a figment of the imagination. But we're here to tell you that chemo brain is real. You are not imagining it. You are not crazy! You certainly are not alone.

And if you have chemo brain, then you're in the club like me. I'm guessing you're not thrilled with membership. But here we are. I'll see you at the meetings. Don't worry about dues. We're all paid up.

PART I

Talking With Your Oncologist

CHAPTER 1

A Vulnerable Time

You find the lump or the swollen lymph node perhaps as you are showering one morning. It has to be nothing, you tell yourself. The fear grows with each test: the mammogram and ultrasound where the technician will not make eye contact, or the body scans and blood work, and the biopsy. Then the waiting. Three days pass, then four. The phone rings, and it's your doctor. Why is there suddenly no air in the room? "I'm so sorry to tell you. . . . " You glance at the clock. It is 4 p.m. and you think on this date, at this moment in time, I have cancer.

It is not surprising that the American Psychiatric Association lists the diagnosis of a life-threatening illness as one of several potential criteria for post-traumatic stress disorder (PTSD). It is right up there with suffering trauma after military combat or after violent personal assaults.[1] Some 3 to 35 percent of cancer patients suffer from PTSD.[2]

At least in the short term, your world spins out of control, and the shock of the news may be almost unbearable.

You turn to your oncologist for help. Now there is an expert in charge, someone with a plan to make you well. You discuss the results of your tests and the type and stage of your cancer. The doctor recommends a chemotherapy regimen and runs through the possible side effects: hair loss, fatigue, nausea, and perhaps mouth sores. But he or she may not mention what could be most traumatic of all: potential and often serious problems with memory and concentration that remain *after* you are physically well.

Needing to Be Heard

Oncologists are the main resource cancer patients turn to when they need answers about their treatment. Unfortunately, many doctors are not sufficiently familiar with the latest medical literature about chemotherapy and brain function, or they trivialize their patients' concerns. According to a survey conducted in 2007 by the breast cancer foundation and advocacy organization Hurricane Voices, a majority of patients reported that their medical professionals did not offer constructive advice or assistance to help them cope with cognitive changes.[3] Out of 471 respondents—men and women diagnosed with any type of cancer—63 percent said they conferred with their doctors or caregivers, but only 10 percent were satisfied with the support they received. Further, they said their doctors' responses were indifferent and/or dismissive 42 percent of the time.

"It harkens back to a philosophy of paternalism in medicine—'doctor knows best'—and even somewhat more perilous, if the physician isn't knowledgeable about a subject, it tends to be dismissed," says Janet Colantuono, who created the survey. Colantuono served as executive director of Hurricane Voices after her cousin, Lois Egasti, founded the organization. Egasti died of breast cancer in 2003. Hurricane Voices now funds school and family programs at The Wellness Community-Greater Boston (TWC). "Knowledge is power. There's really nothing you can do to avoid hair loss, but if you know it's going to happen, you can prepare for it," she says. "You may or may not get nauseous, but it is helpful to know you can choose to have medical or nonpharmaceutical-based interventions to help ease your discomfort. So that's why you would want to have a conversation about cognitive changes associated with cancer treatment with your doctor. Once you know what to expect, you can decide how to approach it. With support from your oncology team ahead of time, you can learn about coping strategies that can help."

Sherry Goldman, R.N., C.N.P., agrees. She has counseled and treated thousands of breast cancer patients since 1993 when she and Dr. Susan Love established the high-risk breast cancer follow-up programs at the Revlon/UCLA Breast Center. Her patients often turn to her in frustration when their oncologists minimize their concerns. Goldman attributes this head-in-the-sand reaction to human nature. "I don't think a lot of them pay enough attention to that literature, and I think they're more interested in the cure rates and making sure patients get rid of cancer than in a lot of the side effects," she says. "They don't want to have to deal with complaints after treatment."

Goldman says that about 25 to 30 percent of her post-chemotherapy patients complain of brain-related symptoms. "That's pretty high, and it is only from those who speak their feelings," she says. And those percentages are backed up by more wide-ranging research. She estimates that only about half get better over time. "They say 'I cannot think straight; I cannot function the same way as before treatment,' and they say it to me year after year after year." One patient Goldman says she will never forget is a young woman who had gone through a stem-cell transplant. "Her memory had been so affected, so deeply affected, that her husband described her to me as someone he didn't even know," she says.

Clearly, people are not getting the validation they desperately need. Some turn to cancer support organizations such as the Wellness Community or Gilda's Club (named after Gilda Radner). Sara Goldberger is the worldwide director of program support for Gilda's Club, which has fifty thousand members in chapters across the United States and internationally. She tells the story of scheduling a workshop four years back for members at their White Plains, New York, chapter. The title was "Chemo Brain, It's Not All in Your Head." "What I so clearly remember people saying in response to seeing the workshop on the calendar was, 'Oh, you mean it's a *thing!*' We kept hearing that over and over, like, 'So I'm not making this up, I'm not crazy, it's a *thing!*'"

Until knowledge about the *thing* becomes more widespread, colleagues such as Tim Ahles, Ph.D., director of the Neurocognitive and Functional MRI Program at Memorial Sloan-Kettering Cancer, will continue to receive e-mails from survivors who are surprised to learn they are somehow *not* responsible for their own cognitive problems. "They didn't even know that memory problems were a possibility," says Ahles. "They make the assumption that it has to do with stress or, 'I'm not coping well,' or they make all these psychological attributions."

Worse, many doctors are not fully disclosing the potential risks of chemotherapy prior to treatment. Some treatments may be more associated with cognitive problems than others, and patients have a right to know. Other oncologists may truly understand and sympathize, but they end the conversation with "What's more important, your memory or your life?" Of course, no one is suggesting that cancer patients unnecessarily give up life-saving chemotherapy. But it is important to get all the facts so that you can make the most informed decisions about your own care. There are steps you can take to minimize brain fog after treatment. So persist in asking questions and gather as much information as you can.

Humor Helps

This brilliant oncologist is actually rather well known around these parts. After reviewing my chart and asking me some basic questions, she said, "You know, it's not really unusual for our memories to give us a little trouble, what with aging and menopause and all. What sorts of problems have you been having?"

"Well," I said. "Last week I locked my keys in my car."

"Ha!" she said. "That's nothing. Last week I locked my keys, my phone, and my emergency beeper in my trunk. And the whole forty-five minutes while I was waiting for the Pop-A-Lock truck, I had to listen to the phone ringing and the emergency beeper frantically beeping, like all my patients were *dying*."

"Well," I said. "I missed my turnoff on the interstate. I was halfway to Shreveport before I even realized it."

"Ha!" she said. "That's nothing. On Tuesday I went to my Wednesday hospital by mistake, and I was on my third patient before I realized it."

"OK," I said. "I accidentally sent an "F-YOU" e-mail intended for my ex to my landlord in California instead."

"Whoa," she said. "Wow. OK. I'm ordering you an MRI of the brain, stat."

Reprinted with permission from the blog, "As the Tumor Turns," by Elizabeth Churchill at http://spinningtumor.blogspot.com.

CHAPTER 2

Rethinking "Chemo Brain"

In spite of the popularity of the term "chemo brain," other factors beside chemotherapy may contribute to the memory lapses and fogginess patients report to their doctors. Among these things are anxiety and depression that come from coping with the diagnosis, fatigue, the impact of surgery and anesthesia, hormonal therapy, anemia, menopause, other medications, including steroids and those for pain, and even a genetic predisposition. Some chronic conditions such as insulin resistance or diabetes may also impact memory. Then there are cytokines, the regulatory molecules in the body that help cells of the immune system talk to each other. But they have also been shown to cross into the brain in some instances and might affect cognition (we'll talk more about cytokines later).

While we often hear and read the terms chemo brain and chemo fog, especially in the news, in reality, these terms are simply not

St Petersburg Library System

727-893-7724
www.splibraries.org

Library name: SPMA

Date due: 8/25/2016,23:59
Title: Diagnosis and
treatment of cancer
Author: Lyons, Lyman.
Call number: YA 616.994
LYONS
Item ID: 32410018222995

Date due: 8/25/2016,23:59
Title: Alternative Medicine
Magazine's definitive guide
Author: Alschuler, Lise.
Call number: 616.994
ALSCHULER
Item ID: 32410017799589

Date due: 8/25/2016,23:59
Title: Cancer
Author: Silverstein, Alvin.
Call number: YA 616.994
SILVERSTEIN
Item ID: 32410015516936

Date due: 8/25/2016,23:59
Title: Your brain after chemo
: a practical guide to lif

Author: Silverman, Dan,
1956-
Call number: 616.994061
SILVERMAN
Item ID: 32410018399132

Total checkouts for session:
4
Total checkouts:4

precise enough to reflect our current understanding of what is happening in the brain. Some medical experts conceptualize what's happening as something like, "cancer- and/or cancer-therapy-associated cognitive change."[1] We don't expect to see this or similar phrases ingrained in the popular culture, or even in the professional jargon of doctors, anytime soon. In our own work, we use the term post-chemo brain (that is, after-chemo brain) because we just don't know to what degree chemotherapy is the direct culprit behind these cognitive problems. In other words, this term enables us to focus our attention where it best belongs: understanding, preventing, and treating cognitive problems that become present after chemo—without requiring us to get sucked into the controversy of to what extent chemo caused those problems.

It is, though, worth pointing out that a substantial body of evidence suggests that chemotherapy, administered with or without anti-hormonal cancer therapies, is responsible for at least a part of the post-chemo brain syndrome.

Point-Counterpoint

Your oncologist tells you that chemotherapy does not cause cognitive impairment and then presents his or her reasoning.

YOUR DOCTOR MAY SAY THIS:

A significant number of people already suffers from cognitive impairment before starting chemotherapy. So why blame the chemo?

It is true, of course, that people can exhibit memory or other cognitive problems before they start systemic chemotherapy. Jeffrey S. Wefel, Ph.D., at the University of Texas M.D. Anderson Cancer Center, and his colleagues found this to be the case in the first-published longitudinal study of breast cancer survivors who were exposed to adjuvant (just after surgery) chemotherapy.[2] The American Cancer Society published the study in 2004.

In a group of eighteen women with breast carcinoma, 33 percent showed cognitive impairment prior to chemotherapy. Then the group was tested again after they completed treatment. At that point, 61 percent of the women showed impairment. Most of their problems were related to attention, learning, and processing speed. When the investigators tested the group one year later, half of the women who showed decline had improved. The other half remained the same.

So just because some people are cognitively impaired prior to chemotherapy does not exclude the possibility that the drugs will exacerbate their impairment, nor that more people will become impaired after therapy.

YOUR DOCTOR MAY SAY THIS:

Precipitous or sudden menopause brought on by chemotherapy is causing cognitive impairment.

Certainly, a sudden depletion of estrogen can disrupt our thinking and even cause dramatic psychological changes. We see similar cognitive changes in men with prostate cancer when treatments reduce their levels of testosterone. But there are plenty of women who are post-menopausal at the time they start chemotherapy. In fact, half of all breast cancers are diagnosed in people age sixty-five and older. At least one longitudinal study has evaluated attention, memory, and other cognitive functions in this age group before and after chemotherapy and hormonal therapy. A significant number of the participants showed a decline in cognitive functioning.[3] So, precipitous menopause can't be the complete story.

YOUR DOCTOR MAY SAY THIS:

Your poor memory is caused by a genetic predisposition.

Everything that makes us who we are stems from a complex interplay of our genes and our environment. We are not simply driven by one or the other. Even if we are genetically predisposed to a poor memory or other cognitive problems, we may need a certain amount of push from the environment to trigger those symptoms. Will that push come from the surgery and anesthesia? The chemotherapy? Antihormonal therapies such as tamoxifen? The cancer itself?

One case in point is a patient we'll call Susan. Her history is complicated. She was diagnosed with attention deficit hyperactivity disorder (ADHD) in her late thirties. Although she had struggled during college, she worked hard, earned honors, and completed a graduate degree. She went on to a successful career as a businesswoman, married, and had two children. Both of her kids developed bipolar disorder, a condition characterized by the dramatic mood swings of manic highs and disabling depression.

Then five years ago in her late forties while going through a divorce, Susan discovered she had breast cancer. It was stage 1 with no lymph node involvement. She had a lumpectomy, radiation, and four rounds of combination chemotherapy with cyclophosphamide, methotrexate, and 5-fluorouracil (CMF) plus antihormonal treatments of tamoxifen.

She noticed a change immediately after her first round of chemotherapy. "I went home, and oh my God, what a nightmare," she says. "I could not sit still. I couldn't sleep. People would call, and I didn't want to talk to them because they were talking too slow. I was cleaning floors and taking a toothpick to everything. I'm not kidding; it was above and beyond anything horrible I ever had." She thinks the steroids she received as part of her treatment may have initially contributed to her mania. Worse, the tamoxifen, a drug that works to block the uptake of estrogen in breast cancer cells, magnified her symptoms, and she ended up going off it within days.

Whatever the combination of factors resulting in Susan's symptoms, neuropsychological testing showed that she had severe impairments in the executive functioning areas of her brain for planning and organization and in certain areas of memory. To this day, she does not work outside the home and remains on disability. Tasks overwhelm her. She loses objects, forgets appointments, and accomplishes very little during any given day. Her speech is disorganized, and she wanders off on tangents without returning to her main point. She forgets what is told to her and has poor time perception. It was her neuropsychologist's diagnosis that "the etiology of her functional decline is likely secondary to acquired deficits in brain functioning, which were brought about by her cancer treatment regimen."

In speaking to Susan, she says that she would gladly trade five years of her life to return to her old self. "To be honest with you, looking back, I would have had no chemotherapy. I would have just taken the risk," she says. "I can handle the cancer. I want my brain back; just give me my brain back."

CHAPTER 3

Q and A With Your Doctor

The Big Picture

Even before unraveling the cognitive issues, whether or not chemo is right for you in the first place is one of the most important treatment decisions you and your medical team will make. What goes into that conversation? In part, it will be your doctor's opinion of your prognosis based on type of cancer, whether it has spread, and if so, to which organs. Factored in will be a discussion on your general health and how treatment might affect you. It is normal to feel anxious during these visits. In fact, some patients report anxiety levels that are so high that it is impossible for them to hear what their oncologists are saying, much less make any sense of it. So, it's a good idea to do the following things:

- Write down your questions beforehand. If you are not comfortable taking down the answers, bring someone with you who will serve as your advocate, secretary, and second set of ears. This is the time to have a person who cares about you by your side.

- Also tape your conversations with a cassette or digital recorder. Your oncologist should have no problem accommodating you.
- Play the tape back later when you are under less stress.

Here are the big-picture questions to ask your oncologist about chemotherapy[1]:

- What is my chance for a cure?
- Will chemotherapy extend my life? For how long?
- What are the major side effects of chemotherapy?
- Will the drugs make me feel better or worse? How?
- What are the nonchemotherapy options?
- Are clinical trials available for patients with my condition?
- What things will likely happen to my body and my brain, *with* and *without* chemotherapy?

If you are reading this book, then chances are you want answers. And, in fact, doctors are ethically and legally obligated to disclose your diagnosis, as well as the nature, purpose, risks, and benefits of major medical treatments or procedures. That is why they often have you sign a consent form ("informed consent") that documents your understanding of what has been communicated to you.[2]

ZOOMING IN ON THE MIND

Cognitive dysfunction is a potentially major side effect of chemotherapy. Here are specific questions—and answers—to get the conversation going:

How likely am I to develop cognitive problems following my chemotherapy regimen?

Your doctor may, understandably, not be able to provide a clear answer to this question because chemotherapy is given often in combination with other drugs, and physicians and scientists have yet to completely tease out the effects of one agent versus another (or differentiate how the various agents interact with the patient's cancer) . . . though some pertinent findings have emerged from recent studies, as we will explain later. Moreover, research in this field is currently so fast-paced that specific answers to such questions may have already changed, even between the time of this writing and the time that you pose the question. So ask your oncologist the following:

Have any of your patients who have been treated with this same regimen later complained of cognitive problems? How many?

Might more than one treatment strategy work well for me, such as radiation versus chemotherapy, or chemotherapy given alone, versus adding antihormonal drugs? If so, how do the potential benefits and risks of the different options compare with each other?

Some studies report that cognitive problems are more likely with high-dose regimens. If you are a candidate for such a regimen, find out what the extra benefits are. What do the data show?

How many cycles of chemotherapy will I need? Is there an association between longer-term use with this particular regimen and cognitive impairment?

What about prescribing one combination of drugs versus another that has also been known to be effective for my cancer type? Has either been linked to memory or other cognitive problems?

Should I worry about any specific chemotherapy drugs?

In several studies that have documented cognitive changes in breast cancer survivors, researchers noted that the drug cyclophosphamide was almost always part of patients' chemotherapy treatments. But cyclophosphamide is virtually never given as a stand-alone agent for breast cancer. Rather it is combined with other drugs. So it's impossible to determine to what extent the cyclophosphamide is actually contributing to post-chemo brain or whether there might be an interaction among drugs. Some common cytotoxic regimens for breast cancer—cytotoxic referring to drugs that kill rapidly dividing cancer cells—include cyclophosphamide with the agents methotrexate and 5-fluoruracil (CMF), or with doxorubicin (Adriamycin).

The probability of cognitive impairment in survivors has been reported to be greater after chemotherapy with CMF than after chemotherapy with anthracycline-containing regimens (anthracyclines are a class of antibiotic drugs used to treat a range of cancers). For breast cancer, specifically, anthracyclines include doxorubicin, epirubicin, and mitoxantrone. Scientists noticed a lower incidence of cognitive impairment reported by breast cancer survivors when the "M" in the CMF regimen—the methotrexate—was replaced by doxorubicin or epirubicin. On the other hand, repeated use of anthracyclines may lead to heart failure in some patients.

In addition to the drugs mentioned above (doxorubicin, 5-fluoruracil, methotrexate, and cyclophosphamide), researchers have found other chemotherapy compounds to be common in studies that looked at problems with language, memory, and other cognitive abilities. These drugs include: cisplatin, vincristine, etoposide, vinblastine, and steroids such as dexamethasone and prednisone.[3] Their relative risks associated with later cognitive impairment, however, have not been well established.

So, for example, if two multidrug regimens are comparably effective for my diagnosis—and one contains methotrexate—should I not take the one with methotrexate?

Doctors constantly struggle to make the best choices they can based on whatever knowledge is available at the time. Certainly the data that we have about methotrexate-containing regimens, though not definitive, are worrisome. Discuss the research with your oncologist, and ask what alternatives there are for you.

Could tamoxifen or other hormonal therapies make post-chemo brain even worse?

In studies at UCLA and elsewhere, breast cancer survivors found to be most cognitively impaired were those who had a combination of cytotoxic chemotherapy plus tamoxifen.[4] This antiestrogen drug has been used for years to treat advanced breast cancer. But in the last decade, oncologists have prescribed it routinely as an add-on treatment for early stage estrogen-receptor-positive breast cancers and to help prevent recurrence. Many breast cancers are promoted by estrogens. Tamoxifen works by blocking the uptake of these hormones in breast cancer cells that contain estrogen receptors, thereby stopping cancer cell growth.

Aromatase inhibitors are another class of antiestrogens that include the drugs anastrazole, exemestane, and letrozole. They are newer to the arsenal in the fight against breast cancer so less data about them exist. As with tamoxifen, the goal of these therapies is to block estrogen. Unlike tamoxifen, which works at the cell receptor level to block effects of estrogen, aromatase inhibitors prevent the body from creating estrogen in the first place. So they may be even more potent.

But this is my life. What choice do I have?

At least in terms of the combination hormonal/chemotherapy regimens, the choice is in knowing that they may not all be as effective as once thought. So ask your oncologist about the risks versus the benefits for your particular treatment.

In 2005, *The Lancet*, one of the top medical journals in the world, published an analysis of several different independent investigations of hormonal therapies.[5] About twenty-four hundred middle-aged women participated across all studies. Among those with estrogen-receptor or ER-positive breast cancer (estrogen promotes the growth of about 75 percent of breast cancers[6]), some women were randomly assigned to receive, in addition to their chemotherapy, tamoxifen given over a period of about five years, while others were randomly assigned to receive chemotherapy alone. After following these groups of women for several years, the authors reported a difference in survival of about 3 percent between groups. About 85 percent of the group who received chemotherapy alone were alive fifteen years later; 88 percent were still alive in the chemotherapy-plus-tamoxifen group. Similarly, for some subsets of patients, a statistically significant but rather small survival benefit was seen among those receiving chemotherapy agents plus tamoxifen versus those receiving only tamoxifen.

So one question you may wish to discuss with your doctor is this: In addition to all of the other possible side effects of tamoxifen— such as early menopause, blood clots, cancer of the uterine lining, stroke, and hair thinning—what if tamoxifen leaves me so impaired that I am no longer able to perform my job or function at home? Is that worth a statistical advantage of three or so percentage points?

Likewise, if you are a candidate for hormonally based therapy by itself, it is reasonable to ask: How much added benefit can I expect from adding chemotherapy agents to my regimen? Knowing that a combination regimen may be associated with mental dysfunction, what is my added risk? Clinical and biological factors are important, but so is quality of life. You'll want to weigh them all.

> *"My oncologist said there are no data out about chemo brain. He discounted it, saying I'm fifty, the whole menopause thing. He patted me on the back, made me feel like I'm an idiot."*
>
> —Barbara, unemployed, formerly worked with the developmentally and mentally impaired. Breast cancer, stage 2, diagnosed in 2005 at age fifty. (Treatment: mastectomy. Chemo: doxorubicin, cyclophosphamide, paclitaxel. Targeted therapy: trastuzumab [Herceptin]. Anti-hormonals: tamoxifen, then anastrozole.)

How will I know if I'm experiencing cognitive problems?
What is important diagnostically is whether what you are experiencing is different in severity and frequency from similar symptoms you may have had before the start of chemotherapy. Statistically, at least 20 percent, ranging up to about 80 percent of people, will experience cognitive problems during or after treatment. The good news is that for a majority of these patients, symptoms reverse or at least get better over time. But for some (perhaps one-fourth), symptoms may be long lasting and debilitating.

Are certain people more sensitive than others to post-chemo brain?
Yes. But it is not as if your IQ suddenly drops from 120 to 80. Generally, the changes are subtle. But if you are a high-achiever and rely

on your wits professionally or at home to take charge, multitask, or recall significant amounts of information, you may notice substantial impairment, while people who are retired or have few responsibilities may notice nothing at all. Sherry Goldman, of the Revlon/UCLA Breast Center, says she most frequently hears complaints from women who are in academia or have other positions where they must stay especially sharp. Just recently, two of her patients left their jobs because they believed they could no longer perform. One was a college professor, and the other was an engineer. "It's a little like getting Alzheimer's," Goldman reported. "And they are afraid that's what's happening to them."

Can post-chemo brain lead to Alzheimer's disease?

There is no evidence of this. The syndrome does not appear to be associated with the same biochemical changes in the brain that are characteristic of Alzheimer's disease. As far as we know, chemotherapy will not cause the "amyloid plaques" found in patients with Alzheimer's disease to be deposited in the brain—certainly not in the same regions of the brain—nor promote the accumulation of neurofibrillary tangles, those twisted protein fragments that fill the inside of brain cells in Alzheimer's patients.

Here is another big difference: Alzheimer's is an unyielding and progressive disease. Symptoms always worsen over time. The symptoms of post-chemo brain *do* reverse, improve, or reach a plateau and remain constant. Also, as measured on objective neurological tests, the memory deficits of post-chemo brain are milder overall.

Another subject of interest is the influence of a specific gene type called apolipoprotein E, epsilon 4 allele (ApoE4). ApoE4 has been identified in roughly one-third of people with Alzheimer's disease.

People who carry this allele are not only two to three times more likely to develop Alzheimer's, but also their average age at diagnosis is about seven to eight years younger than others without it. Researchers have wondered what the neuropsychological effects of chemotherapy might be in people who carry this gene.

That question was addressed in 2003 when Tim A. Ahles, Ph.D., then at Dartmouth Medical School (now at Memorial Sloan-Kettering Cancer Center), Andrew J. Saykin, Psy.D., at Dartmouth, and colleagues reported on patients who were long-term breast cancer and lymphoma survivors who carried this gene and were treated with standard dose chemotherapy. What the scientists found was that survivors who carried at least one ApoE4 allele (determined through a simple blood test) scored lower in visual memory, spatial ability, and psychomotor functioning as compared to survivors who did not carry the allele. There were no group differences in fatigue, depression, or anxiety. They concluded that the E4 allele potentially could be used as a genetic marker to identify who might be more vulnerable to chemotherapy-induced cognitive decline.[7]

So people who carry the E4 allele may be at higher risk for developing both Alzheimer's disease and cognitive problems from chemotherapy. But there is no established connection for those who do not carry this gene.

But I already suffer from some dementia. Will post-chemo brain push me over the edge?
Someone who already has cognitive deficits or may be experiencing early Alzheimer's disease may be more vulnerable to the effects of chemotherapy on the brain than somebody who is at the peak of mental prowess.

A large group of studies refers to a concept called "cognitive reserve hypothesis." The idea is that two people with similar biochemical damage to their brains may have dramatically different deficits. In fact, brain PET scans (positron emission tomography) of highly educated people who are suffering from dementia will often show far more damage than the scans of others who have little education and comparable dementia. In other words, mental reserves kick in for highly educated people, so they show less severe symptoms for a longer period of time. But for most people who develop cognitive problems related to their disease and treatment, those changes are not clinical dementia.

Are there unique concerns for people who are older?

Yes, and several issues intersect. Age alone is a risk factor for a number of diseases besides cancer, including heart disease and diabetes. So doctors need to factor in other conditions and potential drug interactions in their treatment plans. Family or social support plays a big role, especially if there are concerns about cognitive function.

Generally, oncologists are careful about prescribing oral chemotherapy drugs for patients with memory or other cognitive problems because there is concern they will not take the pills as prescribed or seek medical attention for any side effects. Healthcare providers may need to teach caregivers how to give the drugs and monitor for side effects, build in support for patients with more frequent trips to the doctor, arrange for a visiting nurse, if needed, or set up help through a community center.

In fact—and hardly a cheerful thought—the chance of developing any major cancer increases as we age, including melanoma, lung, colon and rectum, non-Hodgkin lymphoma, leukemia, and in men, prostate.

For breast cancer, about half of all new cases are diagnosed in women older than age sixty-five (men get breast cancer, too, although it's rare).[8] Yet older women may feel almost invisible. Healthcare providers are less likely to screen them, offer them cutting-edge adjuvant treatments or breast conservation, or consider them for clinical trials.[9] They may also run a higher risk of developing cardiac side effects from the anthracycline group of chemotherapy drugs (doxorubicin is in this group). As mentioned, the potential for heart problems associated with anthracyclines is well established. But in one study of several thousand women who received these drugs, women ages sixty-six to seventy had significantly higher rates of congestive heart failure than their younger counterparts.[10]

For both men and women in this age group, the type of treatment they are willing to endure has its limits if it takes away their physical and mental independence. A few years back, Terri R. Fried, M.D. of Yale University School of Medicine, and colleagues administered a questionnaire to 226 adults, who were sixty years of age or older, about their preferences with regard to life-sustaining treatment. Each had a limited life expectancy due to cancer, congestive heart failure, or chronic obstructive pulmonary disease. When asked theoretically to choose between either a limited amount of treatment—including a few days of hospitalization, intravenous antibiotics, and oxygen supplementation—that would restore them to their current state of health, or choose the option of no treatment at all that would result in death, about 99 percent chose treatment. But then they were asked what they would do if the same type of treatment resulted in their survival but with severe impairment. About 75 percent said they would refuse treatment if it left them functionally impaired. About 90 percent said they would refuse it if it left them cognitively impaired.[11] Obviously, we need to be doing a lot more to validate and address the concerns of older patients.

> *"I was halfway through my chemo regimen, and I felt dull, like I was not running on all cylinders. My oncologist said, 'Well, we'll put you on an antidepressant; that should take care of everything.' I was so totally taken aback. My immediate remark was, 'I am not crazy or deeply depressed.'"*
>
> —Jessica, an office manager for county government officials. Breast cancer, diagnosed in 1993 at age forty-six. (Treatment: double mastectomy. Chemo: doxorubicin.)

Can chemotherapy cause depression?

If you have been diagnosed with cancer, then chances are good that you have experienced at least some depression. Hearing that you have a potentially life-threatening illness would rock anyone's world. But now research is emerging that may correlate chemotherapy to depression. We know from PET scans that there are changes in brain metabolism associated with how depressed someone might be. In our own studies at UCLA, evaluating breast cancer survivors who have been treated with chemotherapy, PET scans showed that those who were more depressed had more severely decreased function in the parietal cortex, an area of the brain that is responsible for integrating memories and sensory information. We observed that correlation only in people who had undergone chemotherapy.

Is it possible to have my memory monitored throughout treatment?

If you are concerned about post-chemo brain, particularly if you are already experiencing cognitive difficulties, consider asking your doctor to refer you to a neuropsychologist for a baseline evaluation—a test of your current cognitive health—before starting treatment. Then, request follow-up evaluations during and after treatment to check your thinking abilities across time.

Neuropsychologists use standardized tests to diagnose or monitor cognitive and behavioral changes. They look for memory loss, problems with attention and concentration, difficulty with multitasking, trouble retrieving words, trouble with reading or writing, confusion, even difficulty with spatial skills such as not being able to read maps that you once could. They can provide valuable feedback to you and your oncologist and suggest coping strategies—or they can provide a referral to someone who can prescribe medications—if it appears you might benefit from them.

I've heard that PET scans can do the same thing. True?

These scans can provide another type of baseline, actually imaging your brain metabolism or how your brain processes information. You would then have a basis of comparison with each subsequent scan.

The most common type of PET scan uses a radioactive form of the sugar glucose to measure how the brain or body functions and to identify any tumor activity. CT (computed tomography) scans use X-rays to create a three-dimensional image of the body's structure. If your doctor will be ordering a standard PET or PET/CT scan of your body for examining your cancer, request that the scan be ordered with the specification that it also include a dedicated view of your whole brain. (Most PET and PET/CT body scans stop just short of this, at the base of the skull.)

But would I be exposing my brain to additional radiation with these scans?

That depends if you're getting a PET or a combined PET/CT scan. For PET, patients are injected with a small amount of radiation. That radiation diffuses throughout the entire body, including the brain. As long as the radiation is there anyway, why not use the opportunity to capture a picture of the brain? Should your doctor order a combined PET/CT, there would be some additional radiation to the brain as the CT part of the scan uses X-ray technology, but this added radiation to the head is a much lower amount than has ever been documented to be harmful to people.

A PET scan to monitor cognitive damage would be similar to the Multiple Gated Acquisition scans (MUGA) oncologists routinely order to monitor heart function in patients receiving cardiotoxic drugs such as doxorubicin in their chemotherapy regimens. To minimize risk of irreversible heart failure, patients undergo these scans periodically, including one before starting treatment. So it is a balancing act. If the patient's cardiac function decreases too much or to too low a level, other treatment options are considered.

The same could be done with PET, but it would be used to monitor brain function instead of heart function. If you are undergoing a six-month course of treatment for example, then a test after two or three months could provide a look at the stability of your pattern of regional cerebral metabolism—that is, the relative level of activity in each part of your brain.

If a PET scan shows declining brain metabolism, then what?
Your doctors will compare the changes in these scans over time. This may be important information, especially if you will be on chemotherapy for a long time. It could potentially help you and your doctor decide if current—and any future chemotherapy regimens—are right for you.

PART II

Symptoms and Signs

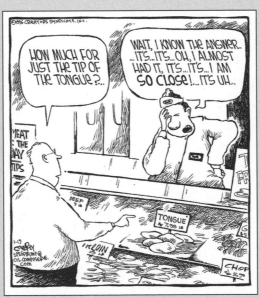

Speed bump Copyright © David Coverly/Distributed by
Creators Syndicate, Inc.

CHAPTER 4

I Found My Keys, But I Lost Myself

It was in 2007 that patient advocate Janet Colantuono came up with the idea to collect information directly from cancer patients who had experienced cognitive changes after chemotherapy. She had just attended a workshop in Venice, Italy, where scientists from around the world shared information about this relatively unknown frontier of medicine. In fact, her nonprofit breast cancer foundation, Hurricane Voices, cosponsored the event.

Colantuono left the workshop inspired but not satisfied that patients' voices were being heard. "We wanted to provide their perspective as a complement to the scientific research being conducted," she says. Colantuono kept thinking about all of the people who had shared their experiences with her. In one breath she would hear how grateful they were that treatment had saved their lives. In the next, she would hear—in heart-wrenching terms—how cognitive impairment had significantly changed who they were, emotionally and mentally.

"I thought, it has to move beyond the anecdotal story," she says. "The *New York Times* would write an article, and they'd have one or two people talking about their experiences. Well, it's easy for oncologists to sit back in their offices and say, 'That's just one or two people; it isn't representative of the cancer population.'"

She knew they could not so easily dismiss hundreds. So she created a survey for patients to report their symptoms online at www.hurri canevoices.org. Other cancer organizations jumped in to help and added the survey to their own Web sites and advertised it through e-mail updates. One of the scientists from the workshop, Janette Vardy, M.D., Ph.D., from the Sydney Cancer Center in Australia, assisted her.

Colantuono hoped the numbers would speak for themselves. Of the 471 cancer patients who responded, all had chemo: 29 percent had completed chemotherapy less than one year prior to the survey; 48 percent were between one and five years out from treatment; and 23 percent had finished chemotherapy more than five years ago. Some 68 percent were fifty years old or older. Most had breast cancer (91 percent). This is not surprising since women with breast cancer are the single largest group of post-chemo survivors and most are older than fifty at the time of diagnosis. The rest reported ovarian, colon/rectal, lung, non-Hodgkin's lymphoma, leukemia, endometrial, or bladder cancer. Nine men participated.

In addition to answering specific questions online, some entered comments like:

"I have had to let go of the 'smart' person I once was."

"My mind is not as sharp as it was; the total effect of all the symptoms is a real loss of confidence in myself. . . . I am not myself anymore."

"My family members and spouse are becoming condescending or patronizing to the woman who says/does stupid stuff or forgets that things have happened."

"One of the most poignant and striking findings from this study," says Colantuono, "is that cognitive impairments experienced by cancer patients alter the psyche. Patients most severely affected no longer identify with the person they were prior to treatment. Contributing to this 'loss of self' is the loss of credibility, respect of others, self esteem, and employment."

Courtesy of Colantuono and Hurricane Voices, here are some telling statistics from the "Cognitive Changes Related to Cancer Treatment" survey results:

At least 50 percent of respondents rated their symptoms as moderate to severe in each of these categories:
- lack of concentration
- short-term memory loss
- difficulty with word recall
- inability to organize daily tasks

Others (137 of the 471 respondents) noted:
- issues with transposition/dyslexia
- intolerance of external environment (interruptions, commotion, confusion)
- fogginess (mental cloud)
- problems with follow-through

Of those who were five or more years out of treatment, 92 percent still experienced cognitive changes. Only 8 percent reported that their symptoms had completely gone away.

Some 62 percent indicated that changes in how their brain works after treatment affected their functioning and relationships at home and in employment outside the home. At home, they reported:

• being teased, criticized, or "supervised" by family members
• children prematurely taking on increased responsibility
• spouses who felt the cancer patient was acting irresponsibly
• not going to social functions due to embarrassment.
• inability to maintain personal responsibility for household or financial tasks.

At work, they reported:

• inability to multitask or organize daily workload
• difficulty learning or retaining new tasks and skill sets
• having to go on disability, accepting early retirement, or being laid off from a job

Frustration was a common theme. Respondents reported that they were frustrated with themselves and that family members were frustrated with them as well.

"Family members don't believe in 'chemo brain' and are intolerant," wrote one patient.

In our own collection of stories from patients and former patients, this theme of no longer being able to recognize one's self, kept emerging. So often our identities are tied to what we do professionally or to how our families perceive us. When those roles shift, we sometimes become like a table with only three legs: We're still upright but off balance.

Patrick's Story

This isn't easy for him. He hesitates, wanting to share his experience yet not wanting to relive the sadness. Patrick is mourning a career that once filled him up, that encompassed a world of intellect, of camaraderie, of providing, and of feeling complete.

Four years ago at age fifty-eight, Patrick was a leading light in his field, a prominent diagnostic radiologist in Dallas with a thriving medical practice. Then he was diagnosed with non-Hodgkin's lymphoma, and everything changed.

Physicians aren't allowed to get sick. They're supposed to take care of everyone else, and Patrick wasn't about to let a thing like cancer separate him from his patients. So three weeks after his last round of rituximab plus cyclophosphamide, doxorubicin, vincristine, and prednisone (R-CHOP), he returned to the life he loved.

"It was way too soon," says Patrick, who specialized in mammography. "But I was so desperate to work. I felt I had to go back." The fatigue knocked him flat, and between patients he rested, head on his desk. After a few months, the gentle teasing started. His colleagues suggested he might have stayed away a bit longer. And Patrick realized he was making mistakes. Lots of them.

"I would lose my place and have to go back and start over with an exam," he says. "I tried to explain a procedure to a patient and I got very confused. The patient got confused. I really panicked when I called somebody I was consulting with to clarify history on a patient, and this person said, 'We talked about her this morning, remember?' But I had no recollection of the conversation."

CONTINUES

Still he hung on for a year, second-guessing his judgment at every turn. Finally Patrick's psychiatrist forced him to face the truth: He was putting his patients at risk.

In Patrick's field, an error could have huge implications. What terrified him was this: "If I got distracted and missed seeing a cancer on a mammogram, then that would have been horrible. I wouldn't be able to live with myself afterward."

He wasn't sure he could quit on his own. So Patrick asked his lawyer to sit with him while he made the call that would end his career. "I'm not supporting my family anymore," he says. "You really feel kind of worthless."

Things weren't much better at home. He could not trust himself in the kitchen. He would leave something cooking on the stove until the smoke detector went off. He left water running in the sink. He got a ticket because his car's registration had expired, and he hadn't realized it. At the supermarket, he and his wife put the groceries in the car, and then he drove away without her.

"We can laugh about it now, but it puts a terrible strain on your relationship," he says. "I'm not the same person she married." The end of his career, the loss of the high-functioning and efficient person he once was, led to thoughts of suicide. His psychiatrist treated him with therapy and medication, and the depression lifted. But the confusion did not.

Testing by a neuropsychologist revealed that Patrick had cognitive deficits in working memory. "He told me they were associated with the medications I received for chemotherapy. He also said, 'It's interesting that in men this often presents as depression because you know you're half a bubble off. The gears aren't meshing, but you can't put your finger on it, particularly in hard-driving men.'"

Patrick says he has finally made peace with who he is now (although he has recurrent dreams of returning to work and getting found out by the board of medical examiners). He takes out a big folder filled with letters from former patients and reads one. The woman writes that *because* of Patrick's skill, *because* he discovered something suspicious on her mammogram and insisted on a core biopsy, he found her breast cancer in its earliest stage. She thanks him from the bottom of her heart. "There were so many patients like that," he says, choking up.

CHAPTER 5

Relationships

Patients who have undergone chemotherapy often mention their concern over how others will perceive them. They believe that people will see them as unintelligent, or worse, feeble minded. Social situations are especially stressful when there is cross talk. "They go out to a pub or a restaurant, and there's a small group, maybe eight people around the table. They just withdraw from that activity because they feel badly that they can't follow the conversation," says Robert J. Ferguson, Ph.D., who specializes in behavioral medicine at Eastern Maine Medical Center in Bangor and serves as an adjunct assistant professor of psychiatry at Dartmouth Medical School.

In fact, a study of the psychosocial side effects during chemotherapy (the same study in which participants reported problems with word retrieval) offered similar observations. Many of the twenty-one all-female participants expressed concerns about social stigma. The women worried about not appearing "sharp." They feared losing friends and their jobs because of it. For them, the cumulative social effects of problems with memory, concentration, processing speed, and verbal expression were far worse than any single cognitive change.

Cancer Affects the Entire Family. So Does Cognitive Dysfunction.

As reported so dramatically in the Hurricane Voices study, some respondents also noted that because of daily disorganization, their children had taken on adult responsibilities much too soon. Others said their spouses had lost confidence in their abilities and no longer trusted them to handle household or financial chores.

Meet Samantha and Mark. Their relationship is strong, they say. But it hasn't been easy.

THE WIFE

Samantha teaches elementary school in New York. She is petite, pretty, and stronger than she looks. She may just be the glue that holds her family together.

"Neither of us is an alarmist," she says. "But when my husband, Mark, learned he had testicular cancer in 2000, we broke into survival mode." Mark was diagnosed on her thirtieth birthday. He is two years older.

"It was difficult. Our son had just turned two, and so there was a baby in the house who had to be looked after," she says. "My focus was on getting everybody through it."

Doctors found the cancer in Mark's left testis. He went through surgery and radiation treatments. Then twenty months later, his blood markers indicated a tumor on the other side. Again he went through surgery to remove the other testis. For the rest of his life, he will be on the male hormone testosterone.

But the cancer wasn't gone. In spring 2002, it spread to his chest. So Mark started four rounds of chemotherapy, including the drugs cisplatin and etoposide, along with the steroid dexamethasone.

Samantha worked at remaining calm for Mark, who had been her teenage sweetheart. It wasn't until each course of treatment ended that she lowered her guard. "I usually got sick," she says. "I got colitis, pink eye, the things you get when you're stressed."

Now, thankfully, Mark is in remission. But the treatment has left him with profound memory deficits. Multitasking is almost impossible. "He gets overwhelmed when things start piling up," Samantha says. She wonders if Mark was predisposed to these cognitive problems and if the chemotherapy somehow magnified them.

"I always suspected, even when we were dating, that he had some form of attention deficit, but it's much worse since his treatment," she says, referring to his lack of focus. "I see a lot of the same characteristics of ADD in him that are diagnosed in my students."

Sometimes she gets aggravated, and then the guilt kicks in. "I'll repeat things to him five times and then find myself asking, 'How many times do I have to tell you?'" she says. "I feel bad when I lose it. But it's difficult for me as the other person in the relationship to keep tabs on everything."

So they sit together and make to-do lists. They sync their home and work calendars to keep track of appointments and their son's after-school sports schedule. And each year, Samantha completes a scrapbook with about one hundred photos of their life together, complete with descriptions. That way, when Mark does not remember where he was for his birthday or where they spent Thanksgiving, he can open the scrapbook and try to retrieve some of those memories.

One area for Mark that does remain intact is his ability to recall the names of songs and all the lyrics. He is quick with puns and one-liners.

"His mind is as sharp as a tack when it comes to stuff like that, and that's the amazing thing," says Samantha. "He has a fun spirit, a devilish glint in his eye. You can always see his mind working."

These days, each anniversary, each birthday is a milestone. "When our son turned ten that was a really big deal," she says. "It was that much sweeter because Mark is here."

THE HUSBAND

Mark could pass for a much younger and thinner Tony Soprano with a buzz cut, and a mile-wide grin. His is the kind that prompts you to grin right back. He swims, plays racquetball, and each year cycles through the five boroughs of Manhattan in a forty-two-mile bike ride.

"I'm very upbeat," says Mark. "I have a beautiful wife and a terrific kid. I live in a really great house by the water; I'm just lucky."

It takes a lot to get him upset. Mostly he is frustrated over his memory loss, what he calls "chemo-nesia." He has mentioned it to his doc, but there is not a lot the guy can do. "He's awesome, my oncologist," says Mark. "But it's like, do you want to complain about what the chemo did to you, or would you rather be dead? It's almost like you've got to suck it up."

Mark noticed the change a couple of months after treatment when he visited his uncle in upstate New York and asked what happened to the uncle's brand-new Nissan Maxima.

"He said, 'I was in a car accident.' And I said, 'Oh, I had no idea, I would have called you!' And he said, 'You did!'"

Mark has the same kinds of problems on the job where he serves as an account manager for a large telecommunications company. He says it takes him forever to remember people's names, and as his wife Samantha tells him, he frequently meets people for the first time more than once. For a while, getting lost on the road for work was a terrifying thought. Then he got a navigation system for his car. "Thank God for GPS," he says.

"I have a brutal time remembering all the features and all the different services we sell," he says. Handling customer complaints or inquiries is a particular challenge. "I would never put anything into my memory because it is like a waste," he says. "I deliberately do not take notes. If they say, 'I have a problem,' I say, 'You have to e-mail me.' Then I can forward the complaint or handle it as best I can." Still, he keeps factsheets with him. "I'll just say, let me look it up. I don't want to give you the wrong information."

Mark says he takes it all in stride because other people have difficulties on the job, too. One of his friends constantly tells Mark that he repeats himself. But the truth is, this particular friend—who never had chemotherapy—repeats himself as well. "So it almost puts me at a disadvantage to say my memory's not great from chemo when other people do the same thing, and I'm polite enough not to mention it," he says.

Aside from his family, what Mark says keeps him most centered is the one week he volunteers each summer at a camp for kids with cancer and their siblings ("Because there's a lot of pressure being the 'healthy' sibling and they need a respite, too"). "I would be devastated if that wasn't part of my life," he says.

And although his cognitive issues continue to test his relationship with Samantha, their coping strategies—that is, Samantha's insistence on syncing schedules, for example—has kept down their level of household chaos and potentially hurt feelings.

What gets to them most now is waiting for the results of Mark's routine CT scans. "I'm always a wreck," he says. "But seven years clean is the magic number for me. Everything is good."

CHAPTER 6

Multitasking, Word Retrieval, Memory, and Concentration

People who have undergone chemotherapy often report their thinking skills have turned to mush. As to memory, what memory?! They grope for words. They can't prioritize tasks, much less complete any. Forget about decision making; it's impossible. Their deficits may lie in specific areas of mental functioning referred to as *cognitive domains*. You or someone you care about may be struggling with these issues. Here they are, described.

Executive Functioning

Think about the roles of successful executives in corporate life. They must anticipate the consequences of their actions (or inactions), plan and problem solve, create and organize information, motivate themselves and others, initiate and follow through on tasks, keep track of responsibilities, make sound decisions and execute them, behave appropriately, and respond quickly to change.

> *"Task completion is where I am most affected cognitively.*
> *It's as if the follow-through feature has been removed*
> *from my brain."*
>
> —"J," photographer. Breast cancer, diagnosed in 2004 at age thirty-seven.
> (Treatment: lumpectomy, radiation. Chemo: doxorubicin, cyclophospha-
> mide, docetaxel.)

The area of the brain primarily responsible for executive functioning can be found in the frontal cortex. (The cortex is the wrinkly
outer layer of the human brain, and the frontal portion, in particular,
is much larger than in other animals.) People who demonstrate good
executive functioning usually have strong connections between the
frontal areas of the brain and deeper brain circuits. Those connections lead to areas of the brain particularly important to memory
and movement control. When those connections are impaired, we
see deficits in the following:

IMPULSE CONTROL

This is where we might see socially inappropriate behavior, such as
rude or offensive remarks, or wanting to kick yourself in the morning for not thinking through how your words or actions affected
others.

MULTITASKING OR ATTENTIONAL
SET SWITCHING

Examples are doing two things at once, such as talking on the phone
while reading your e-mail, or monitoring rice simmering on the
stove while watching TV. There must be enough flexibility in your
thinking to be able to move back and forth between different tasks.

"Before the treatment, I was able to multitask (getting the kids ready for school, working, housework, etc.), but now when there's multiple tasks to do, I feel overwhelmed and just need to sit a little while to figure out where to start."
—Lori, former elementary school teacher. Breast cancer, stage 2, diagnosed in 2006 at age thirty-nine. (Treatment: bilateral mastectomies. Chemo: cyclophosphamide, doxorubicin, docetaxel.)

INFORMATION RETRIEVAL

We store data in many places in the brain, in many different forms and representations. Sometimes people with problems in executive functioning do not manage or retrieve information well. We may not be able to demonstrate what we know, even if we have mastered the material. The good news is that the information is still "in there somewhere," so if we improve or restore our executive function, we will find those memories again. As you will see, brain imaging in some post-chemo patients can actually reveal impaired connections.

Information Processing Speed

This is another area of concern for some people who have had chemotherapy. Think of the speed at which your mental processor runs, or how fast you process information as it relates to movement (psycho-motor). You may not be making mistakes (although some do say they are more error prone), but you are just s-l-o-w-e-r at figuring things out. Everything takes longer. Examples might involve copying figures from one page to another, or typing out handwritten notes, or writing down that phone number, or following a recipe. Processing speed may also affect word retrieval, a task of both executive functioning and language.

Language

This function of the brain is devoted to comprehending language, to producing it verbally, to thinking of the right words to say, and to writing. It encompasses your syntax and how you use verbs and nouns in a sentence. Fluency is part of it—how quickly you think of words and say them.

Word retrieval problems commonly occur in people who have brain fog. If someone reminded you of a word you knew, you would recognize it. But you might not be able to pull it up on your own.

> *"It is painful when people look at me with confusion while I am trying to talk. I know that I'm not making sense, and I don't know how else to talk. When it happens, I die a million deaths and feel very dumb."*
> —Jackson Hunsicker, TV and film director, writer, and editor. Diagnosed in 2000 at age fifty-one, breast cancer. (Treatment: lumpectomy and radiation. Chemo: cyclophosphamide, doxurubicin and paclitaxel.)

In fact, there is actually a "tip of the tongue" state that affects everyone from time to time.[1] The frustration is almost palpable. You *know* that you know the word, and you probably can almost see some of the letters in it. You may even hear how many syllables are in it and where the stress or accent falls. You have a good sense of the beginning or ending sounds (I know it has a "cha" or a "ka"), but the middle part is what drives you nuts.

In a 2006 study of the psychosocial side effects experienced by twenty-one women undergoing chemotherapy for breast cancer, participants reported disruptions in word finding or naming, and articulation.[2] One described this difficulty as "almost like a thought stutter. . . . " In one part of the study where researchers administered a cognitive function screening, language (i.e., fluency, verbal repetition, reading, and writing to dictation) was the most severely affected, followed by memory.

In the experience of Dr. Ferguson of Eastern Maine Medical Center, the most prominent complaint among people who have had chemotherapy is the struggle to recall or retrieve words. So after collaborating with other behavioral psychologists, he designed a pilot study aimed at helping former breast cancer patients with these and other cognitive deficits. The program is called Memory and Attention Adaptation Training (MAAT), and he continues to use it successfully in his practice.

The women in the pilot study had completed chemotherapy an average of eight years prior with either stage 1 or 2 breast cancer. Each had entered the study to learn strategies that would help them with the cognitive dysfunction that still shadowed their daily lives.

One participant was in particular distress. She worked as an instructor at a professional school, and while lecturing to her class she would go blank on the next word or concept. She was fully engaged with the class but simply could not retrieve the word. Together, she and Ferguson came up with an approach. The woman applied the classic Socratic method—teaching not by telling, but by asking questions and letting the students learn by answering the questions themselves. When her lecture brought her to a cold stop, she would ask the class: "What is the term I am thinking of?" Or "What do you think I mean by that?" "We all do this naturally, but she did it in a way to help the students, and she was actually more confident," he says.

What Ferguson found in his research is that those who described these complaints tended to be high functioning. "Our thinking is— this is a little bit of speculation—that these folks maybe didn't have to rely upon mnemonics and other compensatory strategies such as writing things down like the rest of us mere mortals," he says. "Suddenly they have chemotherapy, and they're compromised just enough under load or under stress, and they have to rely on these things, and it's very interfering."

Attention

> *"I'd make mistakes like putting the milk in the trash and the grocery bag in the refrigerator. In the morning, when I was getting some cereal, I'd wonder why a bag was in the refrigerator and assume I had forgotten the milk."*
> —Richard, Nashville, Tennessee. Melanoma recurrence, stage 3, diagnosed in 2006 at age sixty-four. (Treatment: surgery. Chemo: cisplatin, vinblastine, dacarbazine and interferon.)

Attention is the gateway to learning and memory. Without it, there is no conscious entry to other mental abilities. There is no interaction with the world. Think of our ability to attend as on a continuum, from people who may have no outward consciousness (perhaps in a coma), to others who may be delirious where attention waxes and wanes, to conscious awareness, to sustained attention. Even people who are healthy, awake, and alert can have subtle problems with attention. If you are not focusing, you miss information. If you miss information, you don't learn it. Learning affects another area: memory.

CAPACITY TO ATTEND

In addition to the basic ability to attend to all the information that comes at us daily, there is the element of *capacity*. Some people can remember seven-digit phone numbers. Others can remember several phone numbers at once, including area codes. So some have more capacity than others.

CONCENTRATION (OR SUSTAINING ATTENTION)

You re-read a passage in a book several times because your mind keeps wandering. You tune out during conversations. You can't hear your son talk while your daughter pops her chewing gum. You are unable to follow the plot of a film. People with brain fog commonly report a lack of concentration.

"I turned on the bathtub, and I walked out of the room and went and talked to my daughter, and I forgot about it. It ran for like forty-five minutes and flooded through the floor, down the walls, down to the second floor, down around our doorway. I don't take baths anymore!"
—Monica, a psychologist. Breast cancer, diagnosed in 2004 at age forty-four. (Treatment: mastectomy, radiation. Chemo: doxorubicin, cyclophosphamide. Targeted therapy: trastuzumab [Herceptin].)

Memory

Problems with memory and concentration are the hallmarks of post-chemo brain. To learn something, we must first register it or encode it. Then we must store it or fix it in time or place and transport it to long-term storage. Finally, at will, we must retrieve or recall those bits of memory from storage.

There are two classes of learning. One is declarative memory. The other is procedural (or implicit) memory.

> *"I returned to work and knew that I could not go back full time. I could not keep up. I went to part-time status and struggled with that. I had to write everything down or I would not remember. I would struggle with spelling words I had known forever. I would forget names, places, and conversations."*
>
> —Carol, former X-ray technician. Breast cancer, stage 2, diagnosed in 2001 at age forty-four. (Treatment: bilateral mastectomies, radiation. Chemo: doxorubicin, cyclophoshamide, and paclitaxel. Anti-hormonals: initially tamoxifen, later aromatase inhibitors.)

DECLARATIVE MEMORY

Simply put, declarative memory is knowing what we know. By paying conscious attention, we can easily recall it in words. We remember with whom we hung out in our teens and wonder how we ever ate the cheese-broccoli soup in the high school cafeteria. We remember the name of the president of the United States and the hugs of our favorite uncle Dave. We are aware of and remember people, events, and objects. Usually declarative memory is what people are talking about when they say they have a lousy memory.

PROCEDURAL (OR IMPLICIT) MEMORY

Procedural (or implicit) memory is acquired through habits, perception, or movement. Recall does not require conscious attention. After several tries, a toddler takes her first step. We know that if we stand too close to a flame, we will get burned. The classical conditioning of Pavlov's dog involved a type of procedural memory (that is, for the pooch).

Different regions of the brain play specific roles in how we store memories. People who suffer damage to the hippocampus and temporal lobe of the brain, for example, may have trouble storing and recalling facts and events (declarative memory). But motor skills will remain intact (procedural memory). At least in part, those tasks originate elsewhere, in the cerebellum and the basal ganglia.

ENCODING MEMORY

Thousands of images and sounds bombard us daily. We can't possibly capture them all. So we filter out all but those that have some meaning. What we choose to encode comes to us through a number of different paths. They include:

Verbal Memory

We place information into our memory when it is received orally or through language. You repeat a punch line that you heard this morning; you can still summarize the plot of *Wuthering Heights*, even though you read it in sixth grade; you know most of the song lyrics to "I Got You Babe."

Nonverbal Memory

Things that are difficult to put into words—such as a golf swing, the image of your grandfather's smile, recalling contents of pictures, or knowing which streets are best to drive while navigating rush-hour traffic—are put into our nonverbal memories. For people with post-chemo brain, nonverbal memory is a particular problem.

But regardless of how we register the information, we still need to store it. We do that through short-term or working memory, or long-term storage.

SHORT-TERM OR WORKING MEMORY

Think of this as phase one of storage. Generally, we hold on to these memories for just minutes unless we encode them in long-term memory. Short-term and working memory are slightly different. Working memory is the ability to not only store information, but also to manipulate it. To spell the word "grape" backward, you would first store the word in short-term memory, and then reorganize the letters. That manipulation is working memory and a type of executive functioning.

LONG-TERM MEMORY

Long-term memories are fixed in our minds for hours or for a lifetime and can be retrieved when needed. For people with chemotherapy-related cognitive problems, it may be the "fixing" and the "retrieving" that are elusive. Imagine this scene: You are given a phone number at work. Without jotting it down, you rush down the hall toward your desk to place the call. But along the way, someone gives you a thumbs-up because your kid made the all-star soccer team.

With that little bit of interference or distraction (actually referred to as "memory interference"), you realize the number has flown right out of your head. This can happen to any of us. But talk to participants in cancer support groups who complain or joke about chemo brain, and you'll find this is a major problem. We know that when you don't focus on something, you are not going to encode it and remember it later on.

But just because you're having problems now doesn't mean it will always be that way. The brain, the organ of thought, is capable of recovery.

"I am quite amazed actually how my body has returned to such a healthy state so quickly—absolutely amazed. I literally feel like I have a normal mid-thirty-year-old body. I am riding my bicycle every day into work, having no problem at the gym, and I feel like I could do most things at the moment. And the effects of chemo brain have decreased, although I still forget specific details and lose my train of thought. My ability to find the right words, remember conversations, and follow directions fluctuates. At my worst, my brain could not take in much stimulation at all. For about ten days, watching a ticking clock from my hospital bed was enough to keep me occupied. But things are certainly improving."

—Cam, teacher and silversmith, Perth, Australia. Multiple myeloma, diagnosed in 2007 at age thirty-three. (Treatment: radiation. Chemo: Idarubicin, cyclophosphamide, melphalan, stem cell transplant.)

CHAPTER 7

Fatigue and Depression

Cancer treatment affects more than memory, language, and attention span; it can also lead to fatigue, depression, or anxiety. That can cause fuzzy thinking. And impaired recall or attention deficit may worsen fatigue and mood, each reinforcing the other in a vicious cycle. If you must work harder to remember or concentrate, for instance, you tire more quickly. People who are mentally or physically tired tend not to process information as efficiently. Depression may exacerbate both fatigue and cognitive problems, in turn deepening emotional distress. The good news is, if you disrupt this self-reinforcing loop so that one problem gets better, the others improve as well. That's why this book deals not only with cognitive issues, but also with mood.

Fatigue

> *"After chemotherapy, I went back to work, and the fatigue worsened. The lowest point—worse than not being able to string a sentence together—came when I burst into tears at the end of my street one morning, utterly defeated by the complexity of deciding whether to take the bus or the train to work."*
>
> —Maureen Gilbert, in "A Survivor's Journey: One Woman's Experience with Cancer-Related Fatigue," *The Oncologist* 8 (2003): 3–4.

Fatigue is one of the most common and disabling symptoms that cancer patients report after treatment. According to the National Comprehensive Cancer Network—an alliance of cancer centers—about 90 percent of patients who receive chemotherapy, radiation therapy, immunotherapy, or bone marrow transplants report this type of fatigue. Some 30 to 75 percent of cancer survivors continue to experience fatigue for months, sometimes for years after treatment.[1]

Patients describe it as "bone-tired" exhaustion, mentally, physically, and emotionally. You may feel as if you have weights on your arms, legs, even your eyelids and may feel worn out and unable to concentrate. The smallest decisions seem overwhelming.

Anemia may be one cause of cancer-related fatigue. In its mission to search out and kill cancer cells, chemotherapy and other treatments often destroy rapidly dividing healthy cells, particularly those in the bone marrow, where we manufacture red and white blood cells and platelets. A protein in red blood cells (hemoglobin) carries oxygen throughout the body, and people with anemia may get less oxygen delivered to their brain and muscles. This, in turn, can lead to cognitive dysfunction. It can also lead to tiring more easily when you physically exert yourself.

Insomnia may contribute as well. We've all experienced a night where an inability to fall asleep or stay asleep left us exhausted and irritable the next day. Some cancer drugs, such as steroids, can wire you up and spark insomnia. And if you're going through menopause, hot flashes and night sweats can further interfere with a good night's sleep.

It's hard to think clearly when you're mentally and physically exhausted. "When people report higher levels of fatigue, they'll have poorer performance, such as with word recall, processing speed, and divided attention," says Dr. Ferguson.

Fatigue can add gray tones to your world in all kinds of ways. You may lack the energy to engage in activities you previously enjoyed, and reduced physical activity may lead to weight gain and a sense of loss of control over your body. In the study of the psychosocial side effects of the women undergoing chemotherapy for breast cancer, patients reported that fatigue contributed to their feelings of irritability and uselessness. The fatigue along with nausea from treatment and cognitive slowing kept them from working full time (about 30 percent were able to work part time).

In a Dutch study of 157 patients who were either undergoing treatment or recovering shortly after treatment for breast cancer, the scientists found that mental fatigue and depression were closely related.[2] Women who underwent mastectomies, in particular, reported far more mental fatigue than those who had lumpectomies. This is not hard to understand since losing a breast—especially for women without a good support system—can be emotionally devastating.

Interestingly, those who started on doxorubicin-containing regimens experienced fatigue immediately, while patients who received a combination therapy with CMF (cyclophosphamide, methotrexate, and fluorouracil) did not report fatigue until after the fifth cycle of chemotherapy.[3]

Depression

"I definitely was immediately depressed. I was self-conscious about being in a wig in a very public job. I was not coping but crying in the bathroom at work and not handling things at all. If anyone was remotely kind to me or just asked, 'How are you?' I would burst into tears."
—"N," former school director, now unemployed. Breast cancer, stage 2, diagnosed in 2002 at age thirty-six. (Treatment: lumpectomy, radiation. Chemo: doxorubicin, cyclophosphamide, docetaxel, and trastuzumab [Herceptin].)

We see depression commonly, not only in patients, but also in the family members who love and care about them. Depression can rob you of your attention and concentration. Some 25 to 50 percent of people with cancer suffer from clinical depression.[4] Doctors diagnose major depression by the presence of at least five of the following nine symptoms lasting for two weeks or longer and they must be severe enough to affect normal functioning or cause significant distress:[5]

- low mood*
- loss of interest or pleasure in daily activities*
- overeating or lack of appetite, including significant weight gain

or loss (a change of more than 5 percent of body weight in one month)
- trouble sleeping or sleeping too much
- others noticing you seem agitated or lethargic nearly every day
- daily fatigue or reduced energy
- feelings of worthlessness or excessive guilt
- indecisiveness or trouble thinking or concentrating almost daily
- Thoughts of suicide or death, or suicide attempts

* Either low mood or loss of interest in daily activities must be one of the five required symptoms.

Anxiety

> *"I have a busy psychotherapy practice, and many days I don't even think about my ovarian cancer. Then I'll hear of someone or meet someone whose ovarian cancer was in remission for years and is now back with a vengeance, metastasized to the abdominal area, and with a large mass. I can't even tell you how terrifying that is."*
>
> —Joyce, a psychologist. Ovarian cancer, stage 3, diagnosed in 2004 at age fifty-eight. (Treatment: surgery, hysterectomy, splenectomy, and colon resection. Chemo: carboplatin, paclitaxel, cisplatin, gemcitabine, topotecan, doxorubicin.)

For people with cancer, or for those who have had cancer, anxiety is often about fear. Fear of recurrence. Fear of metastases. Fear of disability and dependence. Fear of abandonment. Fear of dying. As one doctor tells his patients, "Don't make cancer your career." That is easy to say after two, three, four, or five years have passed, when the cancer beast remains asleep and out of sight. Because then something marvelous happens. The cancer career goes AWOL. One day you realize with a start that an entire twenty-four hours have passed and you have not thought of cancer even once. Those are the dread-free moments of normalcy.

That does not happen for everyone. For some people, the cancer career sticks around. There is no retirement, no holiday, no day off. Your symptoms of anxiety might range from mild to severe, from infrequent to chronic. You might experience heart palpitations, shortness of breath, trembling, heartburn, sweating, even a feeling of suffocation. You might lose your ability to concentrate or to recall information. Decision making might seem impossible. But as you'll see in Parts IV and V, there are techniques and remedies that can help you master those fears and lessen or prevent their impact.

CHAPTER 8

Measuring Forgetfulness

> *"I noticed after my second round of chemo that I was*
> *having memory problems. I felt 'fuzzy' and had difficulty*
> *staying focused. My doctor said that it was stress and the*
> *medications, and when I had finished my treatments,*
> *it would get better. It's been seven years, and I'm still*
> *waiting."*
>
> —Carol, former X-ray technician. Breast cancer, stage 2, diagnosed in 2001
> at age forty-four. (Treatment: bilateral mastectomies, radiation. Chemo:
> doxorubicin, cyclophoshamide, and paclitaxel. Antihormonals: initially
> tamoxifen, later aromatase inhibitors.)

What the Neuropsychologists Say

When you walk into a clinical neuropsychologist's office, you can
expect to find a licensed psychologist with an expertise in assessing

how behavior and skills or memory and thinking relate to brain functioning. Most likely you'll tackle a battery of paper-and-pencil and computerized tests, each lasting anywhere from two or three minutes, up to forty minutes. You may be there for three to six hours. When you return for results, the specialist will have a picture of your general intellect, your ability to attend and concentrate and learn and remember. This person will also have a sense of your executive functioning, including how you reason, solve problems, and sequence information. He'll be able to quantify your language, motor and sensory, and visual-spatial or perception skills, and he will assess your mood and personality.

And even though you'll probably tell the doctor right off if your frustrations involve attention and memory, there may be a whole lot more to the story. Patients often report more of a deficit than actually shows up in neuropsychological evaluations. In other words, there can be a mismatch between what patients *say* they are experiencing and how they score on the actual tests. You could be concerned about your memory, yet perform in the normal range on a memory task. That could mean the testing is limited or not sensitive enough to pick up subtle differences in brain functioning that may be apparent only under "real-world" conditions. There's no question that the testing environment is artificial; the room is quiet, with no distractions. The typical neuropsychological evaluation is not set up to look at someone's complicated world where talking on a cell phone, taking notes, and keeping an eye on your staff at work happen simultaneously.

COGNITIVE IMPAIRMENT OR DEPRESSION?

One of the first things Christina A. Meyers, Ph.D., looks for when patients come into her office is if they are actually suffering primarily from depression or severe fatigue, rather than cognitive impairment. In the past twenty-four years, Meyers, a professor of neuropsychology at the University of Texas MD Anderson Cancer Center, has evaluated thousands of cancer patients who have been referred to her by their oncologists. "It's sort of like a diagnosis of exclusion," she says. "We make sure it is nothing else, and then we have a correct plan of attack." If depression is clouding thinking abilities, Meyers might suggest the patient consider psychotherapy or antidepressant therapy. If concentration problems are really due to severe fatigue, she might suggest a stimulant or find ways to treat the person's sleep disturbance.

How many of the patients who come to her are actually suffering from cancer-related cognitive impairment? More than 60 percent she says. "And they are not imagining it," says Meyers. How many of that 60 percent get better over time? Half, she estimates.

Neuropsychologist Steven Castellon, Ph.D., also sees people with a wide range of cognitive deficits. Over the last several years he has evaluated the cognitive functioning of cancer patients who come to him through his work at UCLA. There he has served as a co-investigator on several research studies that assess the effects of cancer treatment on cognition. He sees others in private practice. Castellon also works at the Veteran's Administration, evaluating men and women of the U.S. military who have returned home from Iraq and Afghanistan with brain injuries from blast exposures and other traumas.

He, like Meyers, believes that mood and emotion can affect cognitive functioning. "I very much agree that there is a subset of individuals that don't ever return to exactly how they were," says Castellon. "Perhaps it was the chemotherapy. Many of the breast cancer patients I work with have also received endocrine therapy. Or perhaps it was the primary treatment of the cancer itself—the surgery to remove the tumor and possibly the radiation to the tumor site." In any event, something happened in that timeframe that threw things off enough to affect cognitive functioning, he says. "But I also believe there is a subset of people that have convinced themselves they have chemo brain," says Castellon. "They have a heightened focus on cognitive dysfunction. This is exacerbated by both depression and anxiety."

THE PLACEBO EFFECT

Say you're convinced you have early Alzheimer's disease, Castellon explains. You hunt around for your keys for twenty minutes, not realizing you put them in the drawer of your desk. "That event takes on extreme emotional significance," says Castellon. "You may say, 'Oh my God,' here it is; here is the disease rearing its head. But that may not be evidence of anything other than you didn't pay much attention to where you put your keys."

The same thing sometimes happens once you give a name to chemo brain, he says. "You say, 'I'm ready to drive back to my car,' instead of 'I'm ready to drive back to my house,' and you think, yep, yep, there it is; there's the chemo brain again." That subtle mistake could very well be due to a change in brain physiology caused by cancer treatment, or it very well could be the kind of thing you did ten years before chemotherapy and never attached any significance to it.

Either way, there is one intervention you can make right now that is within your control and might also help. "That is, don't beat yourself up," says Castellon. "When you find yourself saying, 'Oh, I'm so stupid, I can't do that, I should have remembered where I parked my car,' try to stop the negative self-talk. The depressive and anxious thoughts occupy some of the same machinery that your brain might better use to find where you parked your car."

WHAT IS NORMAL?

The word is difficult to define, Castellon continues, especially when we're not sure where you started cognitively. For example, if you took a hundred people who have had absolutely nothing happen to them and have no reason to have any cognitive dysfunction, and are as healthy as can be, and you give them a battery of twenty or thirty tests, they too will show a pattern of relative strengths and weaknesses. Some will have no problem taking a very logical approach to things, others will. Some will be better with verbal material, others more visually oriented—we are not all good at absolutely everything we do. We see this in the careers and lifestyles we choose for ourselves.

But some people experience a *change* in their cognitive abilities that dramatically affects their lives. So neuropsychologists will look at their *patterns* of performance. Those patterns help them identify what "normal functioning" means for a particular individual. It's a process that is part art and part science. For example, prior to cancer treatment you may have been someone who would have scored in the ninetieth percentile on a test of verbal memory. But after treatment you're performing at the fiftieth percentile. If someone does not know you, scoring in the fiftieth percentile might look perfectly fine (you would be doing better than fifty out of one hundred people). But, in fact, it represents a dramatic decline that is likely to be very obvious to you, especially if your career or home life depends on a quick mind. So having a good idea of where a person was functioning prior to cancer treatment is important. Educational and occupational accomplishments are ways to estimate pretreatment functioning, but there are also aspects of overall IQ that don't change a lot with brain injury, says Castellon. Even in the early stages of Alzheimer's disease, many cognitive functions will remain fairly normal. "By accounting for the person's basic overall intellectual functioning, I can get a pretty good idea if there has been meaningful deterioration," he says. "If I know that person's overall intellectual functioning is in the ninetieth percentile, then that fiftieth percentile score on verbal memory tasks is almost surely a drop."

Testing can also establish a baseline before starting cancer treatment. At intervals after treatment, patients often return for retesting to see if scores on tasks have changed. If so, that would be a good reason to get help with those deficiencies or challenge themselves with cognitive exercises.

Does Castellon consider post-chemo changes a type of brain injury? "With the breast cancer patients I typically work with, many of the chemotherapy agents don't effectively cross the blood-brain barrier and directly injure the brain," he says. "But could they cause indirect injury through immune system dysfunction, or vascular injury? I would say yes."

WHICH COGNITIVE SKILLS ARE AFFECTED MOST?

What Meyers sees primarily in testing patients are problems with memory retrieval, not memory storage. Her patients describe themselves as forgetful because they go blank when trying to remember someone's name or words or conversation. But they are able to recall the information later. "So it's not like they are losing memory like you would see in Alzheimer's disease," she says. "But they are not efficient at pulling things out from their memory stores." Many also show less working memory capacity, that is, they can't take in a flood of information at once. For example, Meyers may give her patients twelve words to learn over repeated trials. Perhaps they will learn only eight. "It's not like they aren't retaining it," she says. "It's that less is getting through the front door."

Denise D. Correa, Ph.D., a board certified neuropsychologist at Memorial Sloan-Kettering Cancer Center in New York City who specializes in the cognitive side effects of radiotherapy and chemotherapy, likes to use a specific analogy to describe these attentional and executive function difficulties. "It's as if you have a file cabinet and most files are there, but they're not in order or they're not labeled clearly," she says. "So you can't find them efficiently."

Divided attention (multitasking) and processing speed also enter the equation. "What used to take them half an hour now takes them two hours. And although they test fairly well, it is at the expense of much more mental effort," says Meyers.

Effects on Daily Life

Multitasking: overwhelmed by competing demands

Concentration: easily distracted

Generalized slowing: missed points in conversations; deadlines difficult to meet

Increased effort: no auto pilot[1]

Castellon has observed similar post-chemo decline in his patients in the areas of processing speed and executive functioning. Patients might still score poorly or lower than average on language tasks or memory tasks. But, he says, there is a huge executive functioning component to memory, as there is for language. Executive functions are akin to the company executive of the brain. They delegate, monitor, oversee, anticipate, and adjust to situations—all functions that are key elements to many neuropsychological tasks. In cognitive terms, he explains, people with good executive functioning have the ability to better organize information, which helps them encode or remember it more effectively. Without effectively organizing the information that we're trying to learn or remember, we can often have a hard time recalling that material on command. So what looks like a memory problem could actually be an organizational or executive functioning deficit.

Slow processing speed and executive dysfunction contribute to retrieval problems as well, and cues given during testing often illustrate that point. For example, Castellon might instruct a patient to remember the words, "robin," "piano," and "green." After a thirty-minute interval, he'll ask the person to recall the words. He or she might remember "robin" but not the other two. If Castellon provides cues that one of the words was a musical instrument and the other a color, that may be enough for the person to answer, "Oh, yes, piano and green." So like the file cabinet example above, the information is up there but not readily accessible.

There is a maxim in neuropsychology that *you get what you got*, meaning that when brain insult or brain injury takes place, a lot of times it exaggerates or worsens characteristics that were already there. "So the person who was kind of irritable before having a stroke will become super irritable," he says. "The person who was a little anxious and a little scattered before developing whatever the brain problem was, may become even more so."

RULING OUT ALZHEIMER'S DISEASE

Castellon says he spends time with his patients discussing not only what the results of this and other types of cognitive tests suggest, but also what they *don't* suggest. "Many patients are worried that their cognitive problems may be Alzheimer's or that something is dramatically wrong with their minds," he says. But the memory issues he sees in people after chemotherapy are not the same ones he sees in patients with Alzheimer's disease. "Going back to our three-word example, generally, people with Alzheimer's won't get robin or piano or green to stick up there," says Castellon. "So when I say, 'musical instrument,' if you're bright, you might take a guess and stumble upon 'piano.' But you're just as likely to guess guitar or violin or some other instrument—the cue isn't helping retrieval. The bottom line in Alzheimer's or other neurodegenerative conditions is that sometimes you never even get the information encoded and stored in the brain in the first place and chemo brain is not like that at all."

ATTENTION VS. MEMORY

If you have a hard time sustaining, dividing, or redirecting your focus, then probably what you are experiencing is not a memory problem at all, but an attention deficit, says Castellon. It could be that you are not encoding information as deeply as you once could prior to cancer treatment. So to hang onto information, he suggests practicing encoding techniques. Rehearse or repeat what you have learned, write it down, try to visualize it.

RESULTS, STRENGTHS, AND WEAKNESSES

Feedback is an important part of the process. "The people I see are not always aware of the issues of attention and executive dysfunction, of difficulties organizing and sequencing, of being easily distracted and how that indirectly affects their memory," says Correa. "So going over the results and clarifying that makes a lot of sense to them and can be helpful in developing appropriate compensatory strategies."

Most neuropsychologists also map out the positive—those tasks where you perform well. That way, patients can compensate with their cognitive strengths. For example, let's say you are a college student and find it almost impossible to take down notes while your professor talks. Further, you're busy focusing on your frantic scribbles, not on your comprehension. So not only are your notes incomplete, but you haven't a clue what the lecture is about. Let's say you also have good visual attention. You might be better off taking only limited notes, taping the lecture for playback later, and attending fully to the professor's presentation.

As for cognitive deficits, Castellon suggests *borrowing* structure by manipulating your environment with such things as personal digital assistants (hand-held organizers) to help with poor executive functioning. These techniques only work, though, when you remember to use them. You will find help with *remembering* and borrowing structure in later chapters.

He also suggests exercising your brain just as you exercise the rest of your body. If you went to the gym and worked out just once, it probably wouldn't do much good. But if you exercised daily, you would start to see results in your cardiovascular health and in your muscle tone. "You have to commit to challenging yourself, and sometimes that means doing those cognitive tasks that frustrate you," he says. "The idea of no-pain, no-gain actually applies to the brain as well. When you work at it willingly, sometimes you start to see that you are actually getting better at a task, and the next time it comes up, you won't be so overwhelmed."

CHAPTER 9

Body of Evidence

How neuropsychologists like Drs. Castellon, Meyers, and Correa apply certain measurement tools to help patients is just one snapshot of the process. How they use them to *study* post-chemo brain is another. Independent investigations like theirs are moving science forward, providing us with new insights to how post-chemo deficits affect the mind.

Cross-sectional studies, that's to say, those that compare patient groups that have undergone chemotherapy to groups that have not, identify differences between groups. Since 2004, beginning with a seminal report by Jeffrey Wefel and his colleagues at MD Anderson Cancer Center in Houston, the most compelling measurements of cognitive changes have not only compared such groups, but also have compared changes in the individuals themselves over time. Usually researchers follow these patients from the start of therapy, sometimes to years after completion.

Most of the well-designed investigations of this kind document some degree of cognitive decline by a significant subset of cancer patients undergoing chemotherapy (although a few authors have interpreted their data as failing to support this chemotherapy link). These prospective, longitudinal, experimental designs allow researchers to more rigorously assess the effects of chemotherapy on cognition. And so, it is worth highlighting several of those studies here.

In Dr. Wefel's study, cancer patients were examined with a large battery of neuropsychologic tests on multiple occasions (before chemotherapy, about three weeks after completing chemo and one year after completing chemo).[1] About 33 percent of the group showed cognitive impairment before starting treatment. After exposure to chemotherapy, that number jumped to 61 percent. Patients demonstrated cognitive dysfunction most commonly in attention, learning, and processing speed. At one year after completing chemotherapy, half improved cognitively. Half remained impaired.

In a study reported two years after Wefel's, investigators tested forty-six breast cancer patients at similar timepoints as in the Wefel study. Of those participants, one group had received chemotherapy. Another had chemo plus tamoxifen. A third group with early non-invasive malignancy had undergone local therapy only. Patients in both chemo groups deteriorated in verbal memory performance. The women who also got tamoxifen further deteriorated in nonverbal memory. Those who received no adjuvant treatment actually improved their scores (consistent with practice effects).[2]

Specializing in geriatric oncology, Dr. Arti Hurria and her colleagues evaluated breast cancer patients over sixty-five years old.[3] The participants completed full neurocognitive panels of tests pre-chemotherapy, and then again six months after completing chemotherapy. One-fourth of their subjects experienced a decline in cognitive function with memory especially affected.

In a particularly long and large longitudinal investigation, researchers retested 206 subjects at one and two years after their baseline evaluation.[4] Half had been breast cancer patients undergoing adjuvant therapy at the time of first cognitive testing. Half were healthy women selected as controls. Following the first three or more courses of adjuvant therapy, more than three times as many patients as their matched controls suffered from moderate or severe cognitive dysfunction (16 percent versus 5 percent). Two years later, nearly one-fourth of the originally impaired chemo patients continued to suffer from moderate or severe cognitive dysfunction. But not a single control subject suffered from decline.

In a longitudinal study of 184 subjects reported by Dr. Sanne Schagen and her colleagues in the Netherlands, high-dose chemotherapy was associated with a quadrupling of the number of patients suffering cognitive deterioration from pre-treatment baseline to post-treatment testing one year later, compared to healthy controls (25 percent versus 6.7 percent).[5] The controls did not cognitively differ from breast cancer patients at baseline. That is an important point. Their similar functioning refutes the argument that those who are impaired after chemo were most likely impaired prior.

In a longitudinal study conducted by Dr. Valerie Jenkins and her colleagues in Great Britain, eighty-five patients underwent chemotherapy while another forty-three underwent endocrine therapy. Investigators also followed forty-nine healthy controls. Subjects took neuropsychologic tests before adjuvant treatment, six months after initiating treatment, and at eighteen months after treatment started. The team reported no significant effects on the incidence of decline in overall neuropsychologic performance.[6]

But the neuropsychologic data actually revealed different conclusions that were not highlighted by the authors. Performance on an auditory verbal learning task ("AVLT supraspan") demonstrated "reliable decline" at six months after initiation of chemotherapy in 15 percent of treated patients. It showed persistent deterioration, even at eighteen months after initiation of chemotherapy in 14 percent. In contrast, performance on this task by the end of the observation period had deteriorated in both control groups in only 5 to 6 percent of subjects.

So chemotherapy was associated with an incidence of deterioration two to three times greater than in control subjects. And again, for any pre-chemo theory holdouts, it is worth emphasizing that the control group that did have cancer, but not chemotherapy, deteriorated at an incidence rate no greater than the healthy control group. A potential methodologic problem with this study is that 18 percent of its "healthy control group" demonstrated significantly declining *overall cognition* in just a six-month period (!). This is a rate substantially greater than typically observed in the age-matched general population.

Most recently, in just a half-year preceding the time of this writing, investigators of prospective longitudinal studies have reported the following:

- Early-stage breast cancer patients undergoing either radiation or chemotherapy develop verbal memory problems. Those undergoing chemotherapy also experience impaired verbal fluency.[7]
- Significant decreases in nonverbal and overall cognitive function occur in women who receive doxorubicin and cyclophosphamide combination chemotherapy for breast cancer. The effect

remains significant after statistically controlling for anxiety, depression, fatigue, hemoglobin level, menopausal status, and perceived cognitive function;[8]

- In a study of 112 postmenopausal women with early stage breast cancer, patients treated with chemotherapy (sixty-one women) were three times more likely to show a reliable cognitive decline (especially in working memory) than a control group treated with hormonal therapy (fifty-one women).[9]

To sum up, over the past five years, considerable data have provided substantial evidence that at least part of the cognitive decline suffered by cancer patients following conventional chemotherapy is due to the chemotherapy itself. As one patient said, "It's a thing."

PART III

Molecules Behaving Badly

CHAPTER 10

The Healthy Brain

Like all of our organs, the brain has evolved over millions of years. It gradually developed from the inside out. The oldest part is the brain stem. It controls basic biological rhythms such as breathing, heart beat, muscle function, and balance. The higher functions of the brain, though, have evolved in what American biologist Paul D. MacLean, M.D., called the *triune brain*, or three brains in one. They reside in a respectful but wary alliance with the other.

Capping the brain stem is the *R-complex*, *R* standing for reptile. Deep inside our brains, we share the same survival tendencies toward fight-or-flight responses, aggression and rage, social hierarchies, and territorial behavior as our ancient relative the Komodo dragon.

MacLean coined the term *the limbic system* to describe our so-called second brain, the area surrounding the R-complex. After 500 million years, the limbic system is still intact in species across the animal kingdom. It is crucial for processing emotions and moods, and for developing instinct to nurture and protect our young. It is involved in memory. It is seen in apes that swing from tree to tree to caress their young. It is seen in dogs that cry when their owners leave for work. Of course, we see it in ourselves.

The outside of the brain is the cortex, which is also called the cerebral cortex. The cerebral cortex evolved more recently but still millions of years ago. It is here where we process reason and speech, intuition and critical thinking. It is here where in a blink of an eon, civilizations built pyramids and spaceships. It is here where our children learn reading, math, and science and where a gentle breeze inspires us to think of poetry.

Over the course of time, our intellectual and behavioral repertoire evolved even further. We have a larger forebrain—the front-most part of our neocortex—than any of the other land animals. Completing an intricate dance with the limbic system, the frontal lobes are critical to our expression of personality and abstract reasoning. We are aware of conscience and morality. We know that killing is bad and loving is good. We judge others and ourselves. We organize and schedule. We create a working model of the world so that we can anticipate and manipulate events. We worry about the future and regret the past. Ultimately, it is *this* area that makes us most distinctively human.

The Interplay of Thought

But how do regions of the healthy brain communicate? Think of a hundred billion stars in the Milky Way galaxy, each firing off electrical signals. Then imagine the same number of cells—called neurons—in our brain. Each is charged with a current that pulses and flashes like an electrical storm as we think and dream and wonder. Every memory of every sensory experience—the patter of rain, the scent of rosemary, the touch of a child's cheek—is encoded in these neurons. It is their job to pass bits of knowledge along from one neuron to the next through the release of a chemical called a neurotransmitter.

There are perhaps a hundred-trillion of these neural connections in the human brain. Each represents one bit of information. Astrobiologist Carl Sagan once estimated that the number of these bits, if written out in English, would fill the pages of 20 million volumes in the world's most massive libraries. Most of them would be shelved in the cerebral cortex section. "The brain is a very big place in a very small space," he said.

What does the brain actually look like? Think of a ball of gray-and-white Jell-O. The brain is roughly that consistency and density. Nerve cells are the gray gelatin. Inside is the white gelatin or myelin, a type of insulation that covers the nerve fibers. Now to make the brain sound even more appealing, visualize gray-and-white Jell-O with lots of wrinkles or grooves in it. Between those gray grooves is where the communication of one neuron occurs with the next.

People speak about the genius of Albert Einstein.[1] In one study of Einstein's brain published in the British medical journal *The Lancet*, scientists described an unusual pattern of these wrinkles in the right and left parietal lobes.[2] The area is linked to mathematical and spatial reasoning. The researchers compared this area of Einstein's brain to others examined in the study and found his to be 15 percent wider. But it wasn't just the difference in width they found remarkable. Einstein was actually missing an area that normally serves to separate two wrinkles in the rear portion of the brain. Without that separation, there may have been a greater connection between Einstein's neurons in those two wrinkles. Those neurons may have communicated more fluidly, fostering more imaginative thought.

Figure 10.1: Mapping the healthy brain—where it does what it does.

F=frontal lobe
P=parietal lobe
T=temporal lobe
O=occipital lobe
C=cerebellum lobe
B=brainstem

Note: While this figure actually shows the left outer surface of the cerebrum, it should be considered as a "glass brain" depiction: the open circles represent points projecting inwards—either more towards the center of the brain (◯) or all the way through to the corresponding right outer surface (◎).

Courtesy of Neuronuclear Imaging Section, UCLA Medical Center.

Graphics and text by Dan Silverman and Cheri Geist.

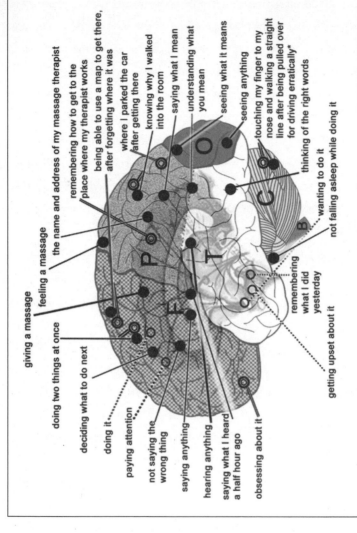

remembering how to get to the place where my therapist works

being able to use a map to get there, after forgetting where it was

where I parked the car after getting there

knowing why I walked into the room

saying what I mean

understanding what you mean

seeing what it means

seeing anything

touching my finger to my nose and walking a straight line after being pulled over for driving erratically*

thinking of the right words

wanting to do it

not falling asleep while doing it

the name and address of my massage therapist

feeling a massage

giving a massage

doing two things at once

deciding what to do next

doing it

paying attention

not saying the wrong thing

saying anything

hearing anything

saying what I heard a half hour ago

obsessing about it

getting upset about it

remembering what I did yesterday

(*erratic driving actually due to trying to talk and steer at the same time)

The cells that communicated in Einstein's brain, and in our own, pass messages to each other. They say wiggle your toe, or help me recall the name of that fruit that is sweet and crisp—oh yes, apple. But they also communicate with virtually every other system of the body. Our state of mind can speed up or slow down our heart rate. Thoughts, as well as subconscious brain activity, can determine if we take a deep or shallow breath. They can express and compound effects of stress, and affect the strength of our immune responses.

As illustrated in Figure 10.1, each of the major regions of the brain plays a distinct, cognitive role. Here is a fuller explanation of what these areas of our brain do:

THE SENSUOUS (AND SENTIMENTAL CEREBRUM)

The back portion of the human cerebrum, comprised by the **parietal (P)**, **temporal (T)**, and **occipital (O)** lobes, is the sensuous portion of our brain. It is devoted to processing all the sights, sounds, smells, tastes, and touch-based sensations that we consciously experience. It connects those experiences to each other and with our memories and emotions. So thank your parietal lobes for being able to feel the hands of your masseur (or masseuse), your occipital lobes for seeing him, and your temporal lobes for hearing his voice.

And thank this back portion of your brain for your ability to remember the whole experience. These structures help us call forth the sounds, sensations, and images of both verbal memories (via the left hemisphere, especially, in most people) and nonverbal memories (via the right hemisphere, especially). We need them for thinking of and retrieving the right words when we want them, and for infusing our words and those of others with meaning (receptive language function).

THE CEO

With our **frontal lobes (F)** we formulate and implement our plans of action. We pay attention, organize our ideas (and things), think abstractly, solve problems, verbally articulate thoughts, foresee consequences, and react (or inhibit our reactions) to emotions and impulses. In the most general sense, we use the front portion of our brain to decide upon a plan of what to do next, and then we carry it out.

To successfully perform this complex job, our frontal lobes must keep a mental model of the world in mind (working memory) and then depend upon the sensuous cerebrum to convey to it not only our memories of the past, but also our moods. Throughout evolution, moods have played a critical role in reflecting what's happening in our environment (is it presently peaceful, or threatening our existence?). The back portion of our brain then selects memories that are most useful and appropriate and conveys them to the front portion of our brain to aid performance of our executive functions.

Have you ever left a pot of boiling water unattended on the stove? Stored napkins in the freezer? Are you lost without your navigation system? Do you regret telling off your boss? Did you run all over town to find the right yarn or tools, but you never knit that scarf or built that shed? Is it hard to stay tuned in to what someone is saying when the phone rings? Blame it on your frontal lobes.

THE GO-BETWEEN

The **brainstem (B)** physically connects the rest of our brain to the spinal cord. It carries much of what we sense below our head into the brain (like pain signals after stubbing a toe). Conversely, by way of the spinal cord, the brainstem sends messages to the rest of the body about what to do (move to the right, jump, keep walking). It also regulates many of the most basic functions—breathing, swallowing, the beating of our hearts, and simply staying awake—so that our cerebrum doesn't have to be thinking about them all the time and is, therefore, freed up to think about less basic (but more cognitively challenging) tasks.

THE IN-BETWEEN

Immediately in front of the top of the brainstem, in the midline between the left and right hemispheres, lies the **hypothalamus**. It drives us to maintain our levels of fuels, fluids, body weight, and sex hormones within tolerable limits, by seeking food, drink, and sex at physiologically appropriate (though sometimes socially inappropriate!) times. Just in front of it is the **nucleus accumbens**, which influences how much we enjoy (and possibly become addicted to) food, sex, cocaine, gambling, and the fruits of our behaviors in general. The front tip of the inside-most portion of each temporal lobe contains the **amygdala**, specializing in emotions (such as rage or fear) that signal when something seems wrong. Just behind it is the **hippocampus**, a structure that is critical for being able to remember tomorrow everything that happens today.

THE COORDINATOR

The **cerebellum (C)** is located underneath the rear of the cerebrum. This structure has long been known to sense the position of each part of our body and then use that information to refine coordination of our movements and balance. (So when you get pulled over for suspected drunk driving, it is this part of your brain that allows you to touch your finger to your nose, or to walk a straight line . . . presuming, of course, that you are not actually drunk.) The cerebellum is increasingly becoming recognized as involved in cognitive activities, though in ways that are not yet entirely clear.

CHAPTER 11

The Unhealthy Brain

So our brains contain a network of neurons that communicate with each other, sending messages back and forth, helping us to do things such as brush our teeth or make a decision about what to have for dinner. This network of neurons weaves pathways throughout the brain. People with post-chemo brain, however, may experience a failure of some neurons to communicate with each other in their pathway. Either the neurotransmitters are not being released or other cells are not adequately responding to them. In extreme cases, neurologists see this in people who have strokes and are unable to speak. Among patients who have had chemotherapy, at least as it relates to language processing, the impairment is much more subtle.

What may be happening, as was reported in 2005 by a group of scientists in the Netherlands, is that the patterns of electricity flowing through these neurons after chemotherapy may not allow different cells in the brain to adequately talk to each other.[1]

A Flurry of Scientific Breakthroughs

In recent years, scientists have made remarkable progress in understanding how chemotherapy affects the way our neurons behave. In 2006, independent researchers working in different institutions released groundbreaking findings about post-chemo brain. The timing was coincidental, but the cumulative impact was to provide validation for multitudes of patients who had long known something was not right. For years, chatter about "chemo brain" had filled blogs and online communities dealing with cancer. Finally the scientists were listening. How could they not? The sound was almost deafening.

Test Tubes and Mice

In a critical study at the University of Rochester Medical Center in New York, researchers directly linked chemotherapy to brain cell death in humans and rodents.[2] Biomedical geneticist Mark D. Noble, Ph.D., and his colleagues reported that three chemotherapy drugs commonly used to treat cancer (carmustine, cisplatin, and cytarabine) may be more toxic to healthy brain cells than to the cancer cells they are meant to destroy. They cultured human brain cells after exposing them to the drugs and also looked at how multiple human cancer cell lines, such as uterine and breast, reacted to the compounds. They found that typical doses of these drugs killed 70 to 100 percent of the brain cells but just 40 to 80 percent of the cancer cells.

The team also gave chemotherapy to mice, and then autopsied their brains. They discovered that the agents killed healthy cells in several areas of the mice's brains, and other healthy cells continued to die for at least six weeks after treatment.

More recently, Noble's group focused on a common chemotherapy agent, 5-fluorouracil, or 5-FU, to see if the single drug would cause damage just like the carmustine, cisplatin, and cytarabine cocktail of drugs. After exposing mice and cell lines to 5-FU, they found that the drug did indeed damage healthy, immature cells in the central nervous system. Oligodendrocytes, the cells that produce the fatty substance that coats nerve cells and enables them to efficiently fire off signals to each other, were also damaged. These cells are essential for normal brain functioning.

A key piece of the chemo/brain connection not addressed by those findings from Noble's studies, however, was the relationship of chemotherapy effects on brain cells with impairments in cognition. A second study further connected the dots between chemotherapy and brain fog. Gordon Winocur, Ph.D., a senior scientist at the Rotman Research Institute in Ontario, Canada, and his colleagues at Trent University in Ontario, injected mice with a combination of the anti-cancer drugs methotrexate and 5-FU.[3]

Compared to a control group that did not receive the drugs, the mice were far less able to navigate a water maze, showing a decline in learning and memory. Winocur concluded that their impaired performance was consistent with the cognitive dysfunction seen in breast cancer patients treated with the same kind of chemotherapy.

In a third study, Masatoshi Inagaki, M.D., Ph.D., of the National Cancer Center Hospital East in Chiba, Japan, and his group used MRI (high-resolution magnetic resonance imaging) to scan the brains of fifty-one women who had undergone chemotherapy for breast cancer. They also scanned the brains of fifty-five women who had been treated for breast cancer with surgery alone.[4] The scientists studied the women one year after treatment and found that the prefrontal, parahippocampus, and cingulate gyri—regions of the brain involved in learning, reasoning, and intuition—had shrunk significantly in the women who had chemotherapy.

The same women also took cognitive tests, and these brain changes showed a correlation with impairment of concentration and memory. In a later study, the team looked at similar groups of women three years after treatment, some of whom had participated in the original study. By that point, the researchers found no evidence of structural change and no evidence of reduced cognitive abilities. The conclusion? If cognitive abilities return, then the effects of chemotherapy on brain structure may be temporary as well, at least in a subset of women.

That is good news, indeed. But not everyone who undergoes chemotherapy snaps back in that time frame, as plenty of patients can attest. Some patients may improve but remain below their normal level of abilities. In another study carried out at UCLA, we studied breast cancer survivors who were still experiencing cognitive problems five to ten years after treatment.[5]

The participants included thirty-four women—sixteen of whom had received treatment for breast cancer, eight who had not undergone chemotherapy, selected as an age-matched control group (similar average age at time of study entry and at time of diagnosis with breast cancer), and ten healthy control subjects who served as a general reference group for comparison to normal brain metabolism patterns in this and other investigations. Of the chemotherapy-treated subjects, eleven of the sixteen had been also treated with the anti-estrogen drug tamoxifen. The remaining five had received chemotherapy only.

The scientists used PET scans to study the brains of all the women while at rest, and again during short-term recall tasks. They particularly focused on regions of the brain responsible for memory of language and visuospatial recall. The women who had received chemotherapy years prior had decreased regional brain metabolism while at rest. That is, parts of their brains were not as active. The lower their resting rates, the more they suffered from short-term memory problems. During the exams, the women experienced a bigger jump in blood flow to some of the same areas of the brain than did the age-matched nonchemotherapy group. In other words, their brains needed to work harder to perform the same kinds of tasks. Moreover, the subjects who had chemotherapy plus tamoxifen had significantly lower metabolism in one part of the brain, in the basal ganglia, than those who received chemotherapy alone.

Barbara's Story

"Although the surgery and treatment were difficult, they were a heck of a lot easier than the fallout from the whole thing. My symptoms of chemo brain were pretty much discounted by my oncologist and the nursing team, so much so that I began to feel as if I were somehow making it all up.

"The big thing I noticed was I could no longer read a book or a magazine or much of anything. I had a hard time reading directions on the back of a box. I could no longer carry on a conversation because I got lost right in the middle of it. And I forget, what was your question?

"I get lost in parking garages all the time, all the time. Now I always park by the cart corral so I don't have to look all over for my car. I'll walk out of the store, and if I walk out a different door than I walked in—like Walmart has two entryways—then I'm totally lost. It's like my mind just closes, just shuts right off, and I'm in a black hole.

"A while back, my husband and I both listened to a Webcast on a Her-2-neu online board. This doctor was talking about chemo brain. It validated everything I was going through, and I sat there and bawled, and my husband looked at me and said, 'It feels good to know you're not crazy, doesn't it?'

"I didn't quit. I went to my general doctor who sent me to a neurologist. I went through four days of neuropsych testing. I felt as dumb as a stump with the memory stuff and cognitive stuff. The testing showed that my ability to learn and concentrate, and my memory have been impaired.

"Would I ever consider going back into the same field? Man, I don't know. I have a difficult time taking care of myself, much less handling those responsibilities and having someone else's life in my hands.

"We survivors need to know that this can and does happen. I would still make the same decisions in my treatment plan, but I would better be able to deal with the fallout of the brain freeze."

—Unemployed, formerly worked with the developmentally and mentally impaired. Breast cancer, stage 2, diagnosed in 2005 at age fifty. (Treatment: mastectomy. Chemo: doxorubicin, cyclophosphamide, and paclitaxel. Targeted therapy: trastuzumab (Herceptin). Anti-hormonal therapies: tamoxifen and anastrozole.)

Gray Matters

In just the last few years, scientists have realized that scans may be powerful, noninvasive allies in the detection and control of post-chemo brain. But not all scans are alike. One of the differences between PET and MRI the way it was used in the Inagaki study is that MRI measures the brain's structure and volume. But PET is different. It answers questions about how we *use* our brains.

MRI machines work by using powerful magnets to measure small structural changes in the brain. By the time an MRI detects a change, there is usually significant cognitive damage. Although cells may grow in the brain following chemotherapy so that once-shriveled regions of the brain look whole again, they will not necessarily function like the ones that were lost. One neuron must communicate with the next to recall memories. Still, recent research tells us that some of the function can be regained when replaced by new cells.

PET with fluorodeoxyglucose (FDG) works like this: The brain uses sugar as the main fuel for its energy needs. Patients receive a small amount of the radioactive sugar FDG. The scans then track the distribution of energy use in the brain by following where the FDG goes and how much accumulates in each region. So as neurons communicate with each other—an energy-expensive process—doctors map their activity. For someone who struggles to recall words, for example, the scan may show reduced activity during mental rest in the part of the left hemisphere of the brain that's responsible for articulating language. For people suffering from fatigue after chemotherapy, we may see decreased activity in the parietal cortex in the back of the brain.

Every time we balance our checkbooks or look for our keys or realize we forgot to defrost the chicken—every sensory experience, every emotion and mood, every voluntary move of our bodies, every single thought that occurs to us—all correspond to some neurons firing off messages to many others. With PET, physicians can often see changes in normal brain metabolism weeks, months, or years before people become symptomatic with any number of cognitively debilitating conditions. The scans are that sensitive.

Tools of Detection

Because PET can detect changes in brain function as slight as 3 or 4 percent, it may be possible to use the scans as a type of safety net.

PET could be used with a scan prior to chemotherapy to establish a baseline of brain function, and then periodically after chemo. If brain metabolism in certain parts of the brain drops by 3 percent, then 4, and then 5, it may be time to switch therapies before the patient buys a membership to the "chemo brain club."

Already, oncologists routinely order PET scans to stage a patient's cancer or to look for new cancers. Breast tumors, for example, consume more FDG than the surrounding tissue. So the tumors trap the FDG and appear as *hot spots*. These "whole-body" scans move from the mid-thigh to about the base of the skull. It would take little extra time or expense to continue scanning to the top of the head and image the brain and would require no extra exposure to radiation from the FDG.

Securing Borders

The blood-brain barrier is the best defense we have to protect our brains from toxic substances. It is actually a semi-porous partition that keeps brain tissues separated from circulating blood. Think of it this way: A group of passengers arrive in the United States on a flight from overseas. The barrier, or specialized components of cells, are the customs agents. They screen each person and each piece of luggage entering the terminal. Like many U.S. citizens who arrive without any sort of suspicion directed at them and are waved right through, the barrier will allow in the molecules that are important for brain health. Those include oxygen, glucose, and amino acids. But like officials who detain travelers arriving without a valid passport or with illegal substances, the barrier rejects molecules it does not recognize, or are too large, or are too electrically charged to pass through.

Certainly the blood-brain barrier should stop most chemotherapy cold, right at the gate. So, then, how are its toxins sneaking through?

The short answer is that researchers have not yet found the pathway. If chemotherapy *does* cross the barrier, it is not at high concentrations. We know this from many studies, including some recent investigations we've done at UCLA, testing widely used chemotherapy drugs such as cyclophosphamide, 5-FU, and paclitaxel.[6] We injected the drugs into the tail veins of mice that had been grafted with human breast cancer, after radioactively tagging those compounds so that we could follow their progress throughout the body in real time, minute by minute. Then we put each mouse in a microPET scanner—a tiny machine small enough to hold in your hands.

Images showed an intense distribution of chemotherapy agent often in the liver and sometimes in the kidneys and the bladder, routes of excretion. We found a more moderate level of chemotherapy activity in other tissues, including the tumor itself. But we found only small concentrations of the chemotherapy drugs in their brains.

Handing Off Messages

The mice studies help us understand chemotherapy's effect on the body. But just what exactly is happening to us as we sit in the doctor's office with a bag of liquid hanging from an IV pole? We watch as the chemicals run through a tube and into our veins. What happens next? The drugs travel through our bloodstreams. They disperse through the entire body. They are taken up by healthy cells and cancer cells, especially those that are most actively reproducing.

But the mystery remains: How is it that we see chemotherapy's toxic effects on brain cells but find so little of the chemicals there themselves? The answer may lie hidden within an unfolding of events, with one chemical process leading to another and still another. Because the brain closely interacts either directly or indirectly with practically every other system of the body, the drugs need only

"I have trouble articulating, I have trouble completing sentences. It's been this way since I got chemo. Believe me, there were brain cells that were massively murdered during chemotherapy. It was genocide in order to get me to live, and I appreciate that. You really don't have much of an alternative.

Here's something that was so painful to me: I had just lost my hair. I had some friends over, and we were playing the board game Cranium, which is like Charades. I got the actor's name Jim Carrey. I just stood up and looked at everybody and had nothing in my brain. These were people who loved me, and it didn't really matter, but I knew that something was terribly wrong.

I have to try to speak slowly and try to backpedal if I can't get out the right word. I used to be very sharp and quick-witted, and I'm not anymore.

How do I cope? I remove myself so that I'm not embarrassed. I can see by people's faces that I'm not making any sense whatsoever. I mean, I know what I'm trying to say, and it's generally astute in some way, but I can't get it out. I assure you that I am not who I was. Admitting it makes me cry, but I'm glad I spoke out."

—Jackson Hunsicker, the editor of *Turning Heads, Portraits of Grace, Inspiration, and Possibilities*, a compilation of photos and stories of women who are bald and beautiful after chemotherapy (www.turningheadsthebook .com). Breast cancer, diagnosed in 2000 at age fifty-one. (Treatment: lumpectomy, radiation. Chemo: cyclophosphamide, doxurubicin and paclitaxel.)

send a message to a cell outside of the brain that then ultimately sends a secondary message to a cell inside of the brain. Let's return to the analogy of the customs agent. The blood-brain barrier is smart enough to recognize the foreign chemotherapy invaders, but it does let in some molecules from the home turf. Our body's own immune cells, for example, release all sorts of molecules in response to various types of stimulation. Those molecules may slip through the barrier or pass signals to other cells that damage the brain.

Getting Better, Symptom-Wise

Just because chemotherapy affects the structure or function of the brain does not mean that patients cannot sharpen their minds. The brain is capable of executing all sorts of compensatory strategies for dealing with impairments. People used to say that you could get by without 90 percent of your brain. While that's not exactly true, functions of certain regions do overlap. When you lose one part of the brain, even surgically remove it, other parts of the brain can take over.

This is seen dramatically in kids who are a few years old and have severe epilepsy. In extreme cases, surgeons perform a hemispherectomy, removing half the brain to prevent debilitating seizures. These children will end up almost completely neurologically normal except for a bit of residual weakness on the opposite side of the body. In their case, the brain is still plastic enough to compensate for those lost functions. The older the person, though, the less plastic their brain is and the greater the risk of serious, lasting effects.

In post-chemo brain there is a much less drastic effect on the tissues involved. Metabolic imaging exams show us that people exposed to chemotherapy have impaired brain function in certain regions compared to others who have not been exposed. But there is no significant difference between the two groups in other parts of the brain. So it is certainly conceivable that even with long-term or permanent changes in metabolism, you will not see long-term, major deficits in cognitive function. Other regions may well compensate.

Physicians and scientists have observed this in people with early Alzheimer's disease. In studies at UCLA and other institutions researching the disease, we and others use PET to scan the brains of Alzheimer's patients. We see decreased metabolism, especially in the back parts of their brains. When we give patients cholinesterase inhibitors (a class of drugs designed to boost a brain chemical called acetylcholine that may slow mental decline) and scan the brains again, we find increased metabolism. It is the front parts of the brains that increase the most consistently.

That makes sense in a biochemical way. Unfortunately, none of these drugs is designed to magically bring back to life already degenerated neurons. But they can boost *executive* function by taking advantage of neuro pathways that are still relatively intact. That is, systems that control other cognitive tasks will chip in to compensate for problems with short-term memory.

So What's the Solution?

Top scientists in their fields are chipping away at answers, exploring how to protect healthy cells while killing cancer cells. Even further, they are using what they have learned from tissue cultures and animal studies to possibly one day reverse those post-chemo brain effects. Ongoing stem cell research holds great promise. Potentially, stem cells could regenerate more neurons in parts of the brain that are damaged and enhance the function of healthy cells. There are drugs currently in clinical trial, such as modafinil, that seem to boost memory and clear some of the chemo haze. More immediately, exercises and techniques as discussed in Parts IV and V can be powerful allies in helping to strengthen cognition.

In the meantime, research continues as scientists see one issue of post-chemo brain with clarity—how chemotherapy affects hormones. As discussed earlier, these agents send many women, even young women in their childbearing years, directly into menopause. Some agonize over the loss of fertility. Others unwillingly enter the world of intense mood swings, night sweats, problems sleeping, and especially memory loss. Those in the fields of cognition and biology understand that a sudden depletion of estrogen can actually change the brain, something that will be explored in detail in the next chapter.

CHAPTER 12

Hormones—His and Hers

"My husband would probably say that his experience with me is different primarily due to the chemo-induced menopause I'm going through. My sex drive is non-existent. And I still feel waves of fear, depression, and anger that undoubtedly affect our relationship."
—"J," photographer. Breast cancer, diagnosed in 2004 at age thirty-seven. (Treatment: lumpectomy, radiation. Chemo: doxorubicin, cyclophosphamide, docetaxel.)

Hormones Defined

A hormone, like a neurotransmitter, is a chemical messenger that carries signals from one cell to another. The difference is neurotransmitters stick close to home, moving in a highly directed way from one brain cell to its nearest neighbors. As we touched on in the last section, neurotransmitter molecules that don't immediately make it safely to their neighbors' abodes, binding to their receptors, are quickly removed from the neighborhood—either being swept back into their own homes by the reuptake pumps that police the synapses, or by being destroyed by roving gangs of degradative enzymes. Both of these mechanisms for removing neurotransmitters play critical roles in the function of our brains. In fact, most of the drugs used for treating depression work by inhibiting reuptake pumps, while all but one of the drugs that the FDA has cleared for treating cognitive impairment due to Alzheimer's disease work by inhibiting degradative enzymes. For patients experiencing neuropsychologic symptoms after chemotherapy, the potential importance of these molecules, and of adequately regulating them, is clear—particularly since features of depression and cognitive impairment are the most debilitating symptoms faced by patients suffering from post-chemo brain.

But hormones, rather than racing to the neighbors next door, take a scenic route and visit faraway places. They travel from the endocrine glands where they are produced through the bloodstream and on to distant sites such as the heart, lungs, or brain.

We produce all kinds of hormones, but there are two major classes: peptides (typical examples are insulin and thyroid-stimulating hormone), and steroids (which include the sex hormones estrogen, progesterone, and testosterone, as well as the "stress" hormone, cortisol).

What does this all have to do with the brain? Well, some of these hormones profoundly affect the way we think and feel. One of the first things physicians generally check when someone complains of unexplained depression, cognitive slowing, or fatigue is thyroid function. People who have undergone chemotherapy may produce low thyroid levels, and that can cause them neuropsychologic problems as well.

The Sex Hormones

It is the study of the steroid sex hormones, though, where science is finally beginning to connect the dots between chemotherapy and certain hormonal therapies and demonstrate how they affect the mind.

The story begins in the mother's uterus, where we all start out with a "female brain." Around the eighth week of gestation, something pretty remarkable happens. If the sperm that fertilized the mother's egg carried a Y chromosome, then a wave of testosterone is released and predisposes the fetus to a lifetime of male-pattern behavior and physiology. Brains not subjected to this hormonal wave develop along the female pattern.

When we hit puberty, the ovaries of girls and the testes of boys begin to produce large amounts of estrogen and testosterone, respectively (along with a host of other sex-specific hormones), and the secondary sexual characteristics kick into high gear.

The Cognitive Connection

It is what happens in the mind as a result of these sex hormones that has interested researchers in the fields of psycho-endocrinology and psycho-oncology. The study of estrogen may be most compelling of all, especially since at least 70 percent of premenopausal women with early breast cancer report cessation of their periods after receiving adjuvant chemotherapy.[1] These treatments suppress ovarian function in many women. There is no gradual decline in estrogen over the course of years for them. Instead, one day a patient is in her thirties or forties and menstruating naturally, and then within weeks of treatment, her body is forced into sudden onset chemical menopause or "chemopause." As if a cancer diagnosis is not enough, she may be struggling with multiple hot flashes, night sweats, sleep disturbances, vaginal dryness and painful intercourse, low mood or depression, and problems with learning and memory.

Maria's Story

"I have a strong family history of breast cancer. My mom died of breast cancer when she was twenty-five years old. She was pregnant with me when she was diagnosed. They thought it was just her milk glands back then in 1972, and they just watched [the cancer] grow until she couldn't move her arm because it was in her lymph nodes, and it got so bad. Believe it or not, she had a mastectomy when she was seven months pregnant with me. She chose not to have any chemotherapy or radiation. By the time she had me, it was too late. I was six months old when she died.

"My two great aunts died in their forties, and my mom's sister was diagnosed five years ago. But she's doing great. I learned just before my diagnosis that I carry a mutation in my BRCA 1 gene. (Statistically 80 percent of women with this alteration of their gene will develop cancer at some point in their lives.)

"I had just turned thirty-two. My cancer was triple negative: not HER-2 positive or estrogen or progesterone positive. People with BRCA 1 and triple negatives tend to have more aggressive tumors. I chose a double mastectomy to be safe.

"I definitely noticed after the AC (doxorubicin plus cyclophosphamide) and Taxol that my memory was terrible. At work, I have trouble multitasking. I don't learn as fast as I did. I know I come across like I'm stupid, like I'm an airhead. I would like to change jobs, but what if I don't remember new things?

"I've never been married, no kids. My boyfriend and I would like to get pregnant. I did go through chemopause (chemo-induced menopause), but I'm told that it's not necessarily permanent, and it takes up to a year and a half for your ovaries to wake up. My hormone levels have changed, and now I'm producing way more estrogen than I was, so I'm very excited. I don't know if I can produce eggs; that's the only thing."

—Maria. Employed in sales. Breast cancer, diagnosed in 2005 at age thirty-two. (Treatment: bilateral mastectomies, radiation. Chemo: Four rounds of doxorubicin and cyclophosphamide; four rounds of paclitaxel; four rounds of gemcitabine with cisplatin.)

From animal studies, we see estrogen receptors throughout the brain, especially in the hippocampus, amygdala, and prefrontal cortex—the areas associated with learning and memory, emotional processing, and executive function. But the question is what is the relationship between estrogen and cognitive function, especially for cancer survivors?

We are starting to discover the answers. By monitoring a woman's natural fluctuations in estrogen, progesterone, and testosterone levels, researchers have been able to chart changes in cognitive abilities. Their work has not always been easy. It is tough to capture that pre-ovulatory surge because it is just one day in the cycle, and self-reporting isn't always precise. (Ovarian hormone levels are lowest when women are menstruating and highest just before ovulation.) So we will predict that the hormonal peak will occur twenty to twenty-four days following the onset of their menstrual cycles when estrogen and progesterone levels are high—the part of the cycle called the "luteal phase."

MALE MINDS, FEMALE MINDS

In the late 1980s, Doreen Kimura at the University of Western Ontario, and her graduate student, Elizabeth Hampson, followed these highs and lows to make a point.[2] Their hypothesis was simple. They suggested that men and women were different cognitively because of their steroid sex hormones. And what they found was this: In women, "high levels of female hormones enhanced performance on tests at which females excel but were detrimental to performance on a task at which males excel."[3] In fact, when estrogen levels were high, the women outperformed men on speed tests of manual coordination, such as correctly inserting pegs in boards. This supported the authors' generalization that women have better dexterity than men. On high-estrogen days, the women were also more articulate than on low-estrogen days. They could more quickly say, several times in a row, "A box of mixed biscuits in a biscuit mixer."[4]

On the other hand, men perform better than women on tests of perceptual-spatial skills, such as aligning a rod against a tilted visual background or cognitive tasks where they mentally rotate or manipulate objects.[5] Although the women, as a group, did not score as well as the men on these tasks, they were better at it when their estrogen levels were *low* rather than when they were high. So if a woman is menstruating, her visual-spatial abilities are going to be better, but her verbal fluency and articulatory and perceptual skills will be worse.

Adding to that, it has been well documented that the right side of the brain specializes in spatial skills, while the left side specializes in verbal skills. So, speculated the psychologists, fluctuating hormones could be influencing different sides of the brain. Low levels of estrogen may activate the right side. High levels may activate the left.

Psychologist Pauline Maki, Ph.D., of the University of Illinois in Chicago confirmed that women are more verbally fluent than men when estrogen levels are high. Maki is well known in the field. She serves as co-principal investigator of two large, randomized clinical trials—the cognitive arm of the Study of Tamoxifen and Raloxifen (CO-STAR) and the Women's Health Initiative Study of Cognitive Aging. She has conducted more than ten other clinical trials that look at the effects of hormones on cognition and brain function. Using PET and functional MRI (fMRI), she has been able to show that estrogen therapy targets the frontal lobes, the hippocampus, and other regions associated with memory.

In explaining the function of the hippocampus—the brain structure in the medial temporal lobe of our brains—she says, "That is what is active right now as you are trying to learn what I am telling you. Removal of the hippocampus leads to profound amnesia, and it is an amnesia where you cannot learn new information." She offers the example of Tom Hanks as Mr. Short-Term Memory on the old *Saturday Night Live* episodes. He walks out the door and crows, "Nice to meet you!" completely unaware that they had met moments earlier.

MENO-PAUSING THE MIND

Maki and others have long been fascinated by how estrogen depletion affects cognition. She cites the work of psychologist Barbara Sherwin,

Ph.D., of McGill University in Montreal, Québec, who Maki calls "the matriarch of our field." In 1996, Sherwin and obstetrician/gynecologist Togas Tulandi, M.D., also at McGill, found that "add-back" estrogen reversed cognitive deficits in women who were being treated for infertility.[6] These women were not able to conceive because of benign uterine fibroids that feed on estrogen. Each participant received leuprolide acetate depot (LAD). The drug suppresses ovarian hormone production so that the fibroids shrink and can be surgically removed. The women went through batteries of psychological tests with scores that were normal pretreatment. After twelve weeks on LAD, they all showed deficits in their ability to recall short paragraphs (logical memory) and to recall words that had been paired with cues (associative learning). But then the women were randomly separated into groups with some receiving estrogen and some a placebo. No one knew who got what while the women were participating in the experiment and evaluation. As it turned out, after retesting, scores reversed to normal in the add-back estrogen group whereas they did not in the placebo group.

"So a woman's natural proclivity or advantage in verbal memory seems to be due to circulating estrogen levels," says Maki. "Although progesterone is also affected by this pseudomenopause, you can tell that the progesterone is not responsible. The add-back of estrogen alone returned them to normal."

PARALLELS WITH TAMOXIFEN AND AROMATASE INHIBITORS

But add-back estrogen is not an option for the 60 percent of women with breast cancer who are estrogen receptor-positive (ER-positive).[7] Estrogen would only fuel their cancers. Most will take antihormonal or antiestrogen treatments like tamoxifen or aromatase inhibitors for at least five years after completing their chemotherapy to prevent recurrence. Others will take it after surgery if they don't receive chemotherapy.

Those treatments, like the leuprolide acetate depot, will also likely spin premenopausal women right into pseudomenopause. But are the side effects similar?

Researchers like Catherine Bender, Ph.D., R.N.—an associate professor in the School of Nursing at the University of Pittsburgh—are finding out. She and her team measured cognitive function in three groups of women.[8] The first received chemotherapy alone. The second received chemotherapy plus tamoxifen. The third received no chemotherapy or tamoxifen. Although theirs was a small study, what they found was that women who received chemotherapy alone showed declines in verbal working memory, such as remembering a list of words after a thirty-second distraction. But they did not show decline in visual memory such as drawing a figure from memory. Those who received chemotherapy plus tamoxifen demonstrated the broadest deteriorations with impairment in visual memory and verbal working memory.

Still, what about tamoxifen versus the aromatase inhibitors (AIs)? Are there any cognitive differences there? Tamoxifen blocks the uptake of estrogen in breast cancer cells that contain estrogen receptors so that the cancer can't grow. AIs (anastrozole is a drug in that group) block the action of an estrogen-producing enzyme called aromatase. Doctors usually prescribe these blockers to postmenopausal women being treated for estrogen-receptor-positive breast cancer because, even though their ovaries may have stopped producing estrogen, other tissues continue to manufacture it. So aromatase inhibitors take care of that. They prevent the body from making estrogen in the first place. In fact, estrogen levels are much lower in women who take anastrozole compared to women who receive tamoxifen.[9] Bender wanted to know if memory impairment would correspond to that drop. She wanted to know if tamoxifen and anastrozole would affect the mind to different degrees.

In this pilot study, with thirty-one postmenopausal women participating (a larger five-year study is in progress), she and her researchers found that women who received anastrozole "had significantly poorer performances on learning and memory measures than did women who received tamoxifen."[10]

Stefanie's Story

Stefanie is at UCLA for an all-day educational program for cancer survivors. The session breaks. She steps outside to the patio, grabs a box lunch provided for participants, and squeezes in at a table packed with friends. What you notice are her earrings—large metallic hoops that flash shards of light in the afternoon sun. What they really reflect is this: I am somebody. Don't mess with me.

That's her mantra these days. Stefanie LaRue will never again trust those who told her, "At thirty, you're too young to have breast cancer." That was three years ago. Now she is a patient advocate, speaking before audiences and educating others like herself. She is profiled in *The Quiet War*, an award-winning documentary about women living with advanced-stage breast cancer. She is active in the Young Survivor's Coalition.

Stefanie admits she was naïve then. She noticed the mass in her right breast only because the man she was dating felt it during a moment of intimacy. "Up until then I had no idea it was there," she says. "I had not routinely given myself a breast examination, and I didn't think I needed to at my age."

Her primary care physician looked at the lump and with all seriousness asked if it was a love bite from her boyfriend. He said she did not fit the profile for breast cancer based on her age, no family history of the disease, and because of the way she looked: fit, healthy, and pretty. "He used words like that," she says. He diagnosed her with mastitis, or inflammation of the breast (a condition more likely seen in women who are nursing), and sent her home with antibiotics.

But Stefanie returned a week later. "I had a low-grade fever, and my hormones were out of whack. I started having hot flashes. My nipples inverted. Now I know that's a huge sign of breast cancer."

Finally after three visits in as many weeks and prescriptions for still more antibiotics and painkillers, he sent her to a breast surgeon, where she fared no better. "He barely gave me a breast exam," she says. This doctor, too, told her she did not fit the profile and dismissed her.

"I went back to the surgeon a week later, crying, upset, frustrated because of how much excruciating pain I was in. I felt it from my breast all the way down my right side and under my arm," she says. "I was bawling my eyes out." In the meantime, her coworkers at the Los Angeles real estate investment firm where she worked pushed Stefanie to demand an incisional biopsy, to get the truth. The doctor gave in, but even then Stefanie had to fight to move up her appointment for the procedure from two months to two weeks away.

CONTINUES

The biopsy came back positive for cancer, and the lump measured eight centimeters. After a bone scan, CT-PET scan, and a full-body MRI, she learned the worst of it: stage IV (metastatic) breast cancer that had spread to her lymph nodes and spine. She went through six months of docetaxel, doxorubicin, and cyclophosphamide chemotherapy, a partial mastectomy (saving just the nipple), and then radiation to the breast area, collarbone, lymph nodes, and spine. "I was given a year to live," she says, reporting that neither man apologized nor expressed regret for the misdiagnoses. She has since moved on to other doctors who have earned her respect.

That one year has come and gone, and Stefanie is ecstatic to report she is now classified as NED—No Evidence of Disease. She remains on the antiestrogen drug tamoxifen but may be switching over to the aromatase inhibitor letrozole. She also takes a number of vitamins and immune boosters, and the nutrient CoQ_{10} to protect her heart, all under the supervision of her integrative oncologist (a doctor skilled in complementary therapies such as acupuncture or in helping with nutritional or lifestyle changes, in combination with standard cancer therapies). "The supplements have helped me feel better in a big way," she says.

But her brain doesn't move as fast as the rest of her, she says. In addition to problems multitasking, the worst is her memory. "I absolutely can't remember much of my past," she says. "Sometimes I feel like a moron." Stefanie is from a small town where most people know each other and news travels fast. As soon as friends from high school and college heard of her diagnosis, they started contacting her online on Facebook and My Space. But she didn't know who they were. Seeing a photo helped, but more often than not she would send e-mails back saying, "Please forgive me, but the chemicals have messed with my mind, and I don't remember who you are or how I know you."

All is not over for Stefanie. The chemotherapy sent her straight into full-blown early menopause. With it have come hot flashes, drenching night sweats, and insomnia. She was told that she could never have children, even if her period returned, because the presence of estrogen in her body would feed the cancer and that would kill her. "The frustrating factor for us younger women who cannot reproduce is that we can't even adopt," she says. "No agency is going to give a child to a stage IV metastatic cancer patient."

As for the man who found the lump in her breast? "We're just friends now," she says. "I would like to be in a loving relationship, and there's no reason why it couldn't happen. We'll have to see."

RECALLING HOT FLASHES

The issue of younger women versus older women is worth discussing, says Maki, because younger women who are on antiestrogen therapies may be even more vulnerable to cognitive symptoms than older women. "Endogenous estrogen in the brain, that is a woman's normal estrogen, helps to maintain her hippocampal function, and it helps to maintain her verbal memory. So theoretically, if you take estrogen away, then a woman's hippocampus and memory will age faster," she says. "That may also happen for an older woman, but she is not relying on her estrogen as much."

That is not to say that any woman going through menopause—natural or otherwise—has an easy time of it. Hot flashes or flushes and night sweats are the most frequently reported physical symptoms of menopause.[11] Men can have hot flashes as well when testosterone levels drop. They are a common side effect of hormonal therapy for prostate cancer or after surgical removal of the testes.[12]

But breast cancer survivors tend to have lots of hot flashes, about thirty-five per week, says Maki. The sudden depletion of hormones blindsides your internal thermostat. Skin flushes, sweating, perhaps even palpitations, nausea and dizziness, are the body's valiant attempt to regulate itself. "They are terrible and persistent, affecting sleep and quality of life," she says. "If a healthy woman without breast cancer takes estrogen, it basically cures her of hot flashes. But a woman undergoing treatment for breast cancer does not have a choice in terms of therapy because she can't take estrogen." Some patients find the antidepressant venlafaxine helpful.[13]

Maki and her colleagues found that the greater the number of hot flashes objectively recorded by electrode monitors, the poorer a woman's recollection of paragraphs and stories (verbal memory function).[14] "What that means to us, especially for women with breast cancer, is that there may be something physiological about what hot flashes represent that is further compounding the effects of chemotherapy on her brain functioning," says Maki.

The Controversy Over Hormone Replacement Therapy (HRT)

If you have no history of breast cancer, do the benefits of hormone therapy to relieve hot flashes and other menopausal or cognitive symptoms outweigh the risks? That may depend on how soon you start taking hormones after beginning menopause.

In what was one of the largest long-term studies of its kind ever undertaken, investigators of the Women's Health Initiative (WHI) followed thousands of healthy postmenopausal women to see what effect hormone therapy, vitamin D and calcium supplements, and changes in diet might have on their rates of heart disease, breast and colorectal cancers, and fractures.[15] Their findings would trigger a mass exodus away from hormonal therapy.

There were two arms of the study: estrogen plus progestin (synthetic form of progesterone) for naturally menopausal women with a uterus, and estrogen alone for women without a uterus due to surgery. Therapy included progesterone for the first group because the hormone protects the uterus against endometrial cancer.

In 2002, the WHI published results of the combination estrogen and progestin arm. Investigators reported an increased risk of breast cancer, heart disease, stroke, and blood clots (although risk was lowered for bone fracture and colon cancer).[16] After following participants for five and a half years, they ended the trial. They told the women to stop taking their hormone tablets.[17] The results were a shock, says Maki. "Prior to the Women's Health Initiative, cardiovascular disease prevention was thought to be almost guaranteed with hormone therapy," she says. "It was almost a rule, but nobody had proved it."

Then in 2004, investigators ended the estrogen-alone portion of the trial after about seven years of follow-up, also for safety reasons.[18] They concluded that estrogen neither increases nor decreases the chance for heart disease, which had been one of the key questions of the study. But estrogen alone appeared to increase the risk of stroke. It decreased the risk of hip fracture. There was no evidence that it increased the risk of breast cancer.

Adding to the distress was an ancillary study, this one looking at the effects of hormone therapy on dementia symptoms in postmenopausal women between sixty-five and seventy-nine years old.[19]

And what the researchers found was that estrogen plus progestin doubled the risk of dementia in older women. The results were similar in the estrogen-only group but less dramatic.

"This was the first broadscale study looking at whether estrogen was good for memory and good for cognitive function as we age, and it said, 'No,'" says Maki. "So everybody was like, whoa, were we wrong! What it tells us is that we cannot initiate hormone therapy in a woman older than sixty-five."

But estrogen use earlier at around the time of menopause may be good for the brain and prevent dementia, says Maki. She refers to this as the "critical period" hypothesis—a window of opportunity when estrogen is neuroprotective. Our own imaging analyses, examining brain PET scans obtained in a study led by psychiatrist and principal investigator Natalie Rasgon at Stanford University, suggest that recently postmenopausal women in a therapy arm randomized to continue estrogen replacement, rather than quitting it, may in fact be protecting their brains from age-related decline and Alzheimer's disease. Early exposure also appears cardioprotective, whereas later exposure may actually increase your risk for cardiovascular disease.[20]

What Went Wrong?

For nearly four decades, doctors had routinely prescribed hormone replacement therapy for postmenopausal women to slow down the aging process and to prevent heart disease based on epidemiological studies and laboratory research, but not clinical trials. But then in 2002, the highly publicized Women's Health Initiative study (using the most rigorous type of experimental design called a prospective randomized clinical trial or RCT) found otherwise.

How could forty years of clinical practice based on established data have been so wrong? Key factors appear to have been "inadequate use of appropriate study design," over-reliance on observational data, disregard for RCTs not favorable to hormone replacement therapy, and poor interpretation of epidemiological studies."[21]

"Gold Standard" Drug Studies

Living human participants—rather than mice or other animals, human tissue or cell lines or computer models or epidemiologic statistics.

Prospective—designed in advance of conducting the experiment. This includes rules for interpreting the data before they have been collected and analyzed and become vulnerable to bias.

Multicentered—gathered by multiple investigators from multiple facilities located in multiple geographic areas. This ensures that the results are generalizable.

Large scale—so there is enough "statistical power" to identify the smallest clinically meaningful effects.

Randomized—participants are randomly assigned to treatment and placebo groups.

Double Blind—neither the subjects nor the investigators know who is assigned to which group.

Testosterone and the Masculine Brain

As mentioned earlier, while still in the uterus, a symphony of events transforms a female brain into a male brain. This is accomplished not only by testosterone but, surprisingly, in large part by estrogen. That's because the testosterone that males produce enters the brain after crossing the blood-brain barrier, and there much of it is converted to estrogen by an enzyme called aromatase. It is actually estrogen that substantially "defeminizes" the male brain (that is, erases specifically female characteristics), while the remaining testosterone contributes to "masculinizing" it (adds specifically male characteristics). Throughout life, estrogen receptors and testosterone receptors co-exist in the same cells in several areas of the male brain that are responsible for memory and learning.[22]

Defeminization does not happen in the female brain because in utero, proteins bind up estrogens produced in the body so that they can't cross the blood-brain barrier. The female brain remains female.

And remember the finding of Kimura and Hampson that "high levels of female hormones enhanced performance on tests at which females excel but were detrimental to performance on a task at which males excel"? Well, cognitive skills for men also may be intricately linked to their male brains. It appears that when testosterone levels are high, men perform better on cognitive tests that favor men. But when circulating levels of androgens are too high—like in people who abuse anabolic steroids to enhance athletic performance—more androgens convert to estrogens. Those men actually show worse visual-spatial skills and improvements in verbal memory performance.[23]

Hormones and Prostate Cancer

Prostate cancer is the second-most common cancer diagnosed in American and European men, following lung cancer.[24] Some 91 percent of all men diagnosed with prostate cancer in the United States survive more than ten years. No one knows exactly what causes prostate cancer, although age and family history place men at greater risk. We do know that androgens (generally testosterone) produced mostly in the testes prompt the tumor cells to grow, once cancer develops. So doctors often suggest hormone therapy, called androgen deprivation, to block the body's ability to use these hormones or lower the levels. Surgery can work in a similar way. By removing the glandular (hormone-producing) tissue from the lining of each testicle, you slow or stop the growth of the prostate tumor cells, at least for a while.

But just as chemotherapy and antihormonal treatments send women into a menopausal spin, the same thing can happen in men. Men experience an abrupt decline in both testosterone and estradiol, the estrogen converted from testosterone. They may experience severe fatigue, low energy, loss of sexual function, and poor bladder control. But findings surrounding cognitive function are mixed. Results of a 2005 study found that "the cognitive domains of verbal fluency, visual recognition, and visual memory were associated with decline in estradiol during androgen deprivation." But researchers in a larger and more recent study concluded that although men with prostate cancer struggled with quality of life issues, cognitive problems were not among them.

Men and Women Adapting

"There is some acclimation to these shifts in hormones, and that should bring people solace," says Maki. She provides the example of one of her colleagues who is a breast cancer survivor and a keen observer of her own cognitive difficulties. For three years after treatment, the woman worked hard at taking good notes to make up for her poor memory. Then the friend announced she was no longer fuzzy headed. "Her body had habituated to being in this low estrogen state," says Maki. "Maybe there were alternative circuits made. Maybe her brain got more adept at compensating."

We can improve our brain function and at any age. What is more encouraging is that none of us need wait around passively for this to happen, as we'll see in the next section.

Part IV

Getting Your Brain Back on Track

CHAPTER 13

Depressing Days?

Depression is a separate issue from cognitive impairment, but often when people are depressed they also struggle with memory, attention, and concentration problems. Clearly, the symptoms of post-chemo brain and depression overlap. We know from our studies at UCLA that specific brain changes correlate with the severity of depression, just as specific brain changes correlate with the severity of short-term memory impairment. Depression is rooted in biology. So are memory problems. Both are forms of neurologic dysfunction.

You may very well be depressed after facing a life-threatening illness, as are 25 to 50 percent of all cancer patients.[1] You also may be suffering cognitive problems caused by treatment. It is important to tease out what is what and treat your symptoms appropriately.

How Do You Know the Difference?

Start by assessing your behavior and emotions. For some people, feelings of depression are short-lived. You soon feel better physically or you regain a sense of wonder in life's possibilities, and like releasing a birthday balloon into the wind, your spirits rise.

For others, the depressed mood persists (see Chapter 7 for specific characteristics of depression). If you see your own symptoms on the list, remember that clinical depression is defined as having five or more of those symptoms that last for two weeks or longer. They must be severe enough to affect normal functioning. At least one of the symptoms will be either depressed mood or loss of interest or pleasure in daily activities. Others may include significant weight gain or weight loss, sleeping too much or too little, a state of agitation or lethargy noticed by others, fatigue or reduced energy, feelings of worthlessness or guilt, problems with memory or concentration, or thoughts of suicide.

Some symptoms of depression can be caused by nutrient or electrolyte imbalances such as in calcium, potassium, sodium, vitamin B_{12}, or folate, as well as by an excess of thyroid hormone (hyperthyroidism) or not enough thyroid hormone (hypothyroidism). If you think you are depressed, the first step would be to consult with your doctor, who may run a blood panel to test for these kinds of abnormalities.

Should it turn out that such an imbalance or condition is the culprit, your doctor would most likely reassess your mood after treatment (for example, with synthetic thyroid hormone for hypothyroidism). If your depression persists, or your blood labs are normal, you might ask your doctor if antidepressant therapy would be appropriate for you.

Generally, doctors treat the depression first and see what cognitive deficits remain. If your depression significantly improves, and you are still experiencing memory or other cognitive problems, consider requesting a formal neuropsychologic evaluation of your cognitive functioning.

If there were anything good to say about depression, it would be that it is treatable. So if you truly are depressed, most likely your doctor will recommend behavioral therapy, psychosocial support (such as a cancer support group), or medication or some combination.

Cognitive Therapy

Cognitive therapy works well for depression. Over the years, investigators in controlled clinical trials have compared cognitive therapy to treatment with medications (and placebos). What the data say is that in the short term, cognitive therapy is just as effective as pharmacologic antidepressants to treat anxiety and depression. Combining the two is better still. But if you have to pick only one strategy, then the benefits of cognitive therapy have been shown to last over time. This type of therapy helps people acquire lifelong skills to prevent recurrence of major depressive episodes.

HOW IT WORKS

The underlying theory behind cognitive therapy is that there is a cycle of events. Your mood affects your thinking, and your thinking feeds back and affects your mood. So if you are depressed, your thinking and particularly your memory of past events will be unduly negative, too. This has been demonstrated in laboratory-type settings where participants were induced into either positive or negative moods, depending on the material they were shown. So for positive moods they would, for example, read a series of sentences conveying increasingly good moods, watch videos portraying happy scenes, or listen to lively, upbeat music. Participants who were in a depressed mood remembered predominantly negative material, and those in happy moods remembered mostly positive material.[2]

The same applies in therapeutic settings. People who are depressed and recount their life stories will focus on all the negative events and give short shrift to all the good things that have happened in their lives. These associations can be particularly debilitating for people who are depressed. Their low moods reinforce the negative thoughts that, in turn, reinforce their low moods and lock in the depression.

Cognitive therapists try to disrupt the cycle of depression by challenging a person's negative thoughts. An example might be interrupting a patient who is over-generalizing. A therapist might ask something like, "Really? That has happened *all* of your life?" or "You didn't accomplish *anything* worthwhile the entire past week?"

Antidepressants

Antidepressants work by balancing neurotransmitter activity in the brain. As we talked about earlier, neurotransmitters are the chemical messengers that pass messages between neurons, a type of brain cell. These messages relay all kinds of information about mood, emotions, appetite, behavior, sensations, and even body temperature, and they pass from one neuron to the next.

The path of information flows like this: The neurotransmitter hands off the message from the sending neuron to the receiving neuron. To get to the receiving neuron, the messengers traverse a space between them, called the synapse. Once through, they attach to a receptor on the receiving neuron and deliver the goods.

But their work doesn't end there. These chemical messengers are part of a great recycling system. Once their job is done, enzymes either break them down or they return to the sending neuron where they are pumped back into the cell for reuse. That process is called *reuptake*.

An imbalance of particular neurotransmitters in that area between the neurons can lead to depression or a low mood. So antidepressants work to correct the imbalance by either increasing production of one or more neurotransmitters or by slowing their breakdown.

The three neurotransmitter systems that have been targets for most of the medications used to treat depression are dopamine, norepinephrine, and serotonin. Each plays a specific role in the brain.

DOPAMINE

Dopamine is the neurotransmitter that is most implicated in addictive behaviors. Drug addictions occur more readily in people who have inherited an abnormal dopamine receptor, for example. It is also a major transmitter in the reward pathway of the brain. Pleasurable activities such as eating and sex, release dopamine, so in terms of evolution, behaviors that promote human survival activate our built-in reward system.

Without enough dopamine, you are fatigued, lack drive and motivation, and find little pleasure in normal activities. Dopamine also controls the flow of information from other parts of the brain, including attention, memory, and problem-solving tasks. People with Parkinson's disease don't have enough dopamine. People with schizophrenia suffering from psychotic thinking and hallucinations have too much electrical-chemical activity flowing through their dopamine systems.

NOREPINEPHRINE

The neurotransmitter norepinephrine is closely related to dopamine. It is also structurally related to the hormone adrenalin (also called epinephrine) and is a major stimulating neurotransmitter in the brain stem. Outside the brain, it serves as a transmitter for the sympathetic nervous system, prompting us to respond with "fight or flight" in an emergency. When that happens, we experience a rush of norepinephrine and epinephrine as our heart rate quickens and our energy levels blast off. Without enough norepinephrine, we are inattentive and less alert.

SEROTONIN

Serotonin is an inhibitory neurotransmitter that is associated with sleep, mood, sexuality, appetite, memory, learning, heart function, and hormone regulation. It is a derivative of tryptophan, an amino acid also found in milk. Healthy levels of serotonin promote a sense of well-being. Low levels can cause depression, anxiety, panic attacks, loss of libido, food cravings, sleep problems, migraine headaches, problems with memory and concentration, and aggressive behavior. Too much serotonin may produce a sedative effect.

Selective serotonin reuptake inhibitors (SSRIs) are a class of drugs used to treat serotonin imbalances. Drugs such as Prozac, Cymbalta, Lexapro, and Zoloft are in this class. Normally the sending neuron vacuums back up the excess serotonin so that it can be released again. These drugs block or inhibit that reuptake, leaving more serotonin available in the synapses of the brain.

In addition to the neurotransmitter systems that are especially targeted by antidepressants, other major neurotransmitters in the human brain are:

GABA (GAMMA AMINOBUTYRIC ACID) AND GLUTAMATE

If the human brain were an automobile, the GABA system would be the breaks, and the glutamate system would be the accelerator.

GABA is the major inhibitory neurotransmitter in the brain. Its primary role is to prevent over-stimulation and help reduce stress and anxiety. It regulates mood and calms nerves. Excessive levels of GABA may impair functioning by sedating you or making you drowsy.

Glutamate is the major excitatory neurotransmitter in the brain. Too much glutamate can be toxic to nerve cells and may contribute to some neurological disorders. Not enough glutamate may impair learning and memory.

ACETYLCHOLINE

Acetylcholine has been especially linked to memory. In fact, four out of the five drugs that the FDA has approved for treating Alzheimer's disease work by boosting acetylcholine levels. So you need acetylcholine for a good memory. Many of the drugs that make you feel better emotionally though (such as tricyclic antidepressants), are bad for acetylcholine levels. They have what is called anticholinergic effects, meaning they block acetylcholine in the body. So they could negatively affect memory. They also may cause dry mouth, sedation, constipation, or problems with urination.

Choosing an Antidepressant

Just as neurotransmitters have specific jobs in the brain, antidepressants work on specific neurotransmitter systems. But finding the right drug to alleviate symptoms is not always easy. At least for now, there is no perfect way to figure out if your depression is based on too little serotonin, or dopamine, and/or norepinephrine. Someday we will have the ability to do so. In fact, one of the promising avenues of brain imaging research, right now, involves the study of individual patterns of brain metabolism or neurotransmitter deficits, so that you can accurately select a class of antidepressants for a particular person.

Until then, identifying the right drug for someone isn't about which drug will be most effective, but rather which side effect profile the person will best tolerate. The SSRIs in general have fewer side effects than the norepinephrine reuptake inhibitors. People often start with them. But most of the SSRIs are associated with impairment of sexual function. So if that will be a major impediment to your life and relationships, then you might want to choose from another class of antidepressants.

Sometimes you actually want a side effect. If your depression is accompanied by agitation and anxiety, for example, then you might want a drug that happens to also sedate. If you are depressed with slow movement, fatigue, and drowsiness, then you will want to avoid sedating drugs.

Here is a list of antidepressants by categories that will give you an idea of how they work on neurotransmitters.

Classes of Antidepressants

SELECTIVE SEROTONIN REUPTAKE INHIBITORS (SSRIs)

These include fluoxetine (Prozac), sertraline (Zoloft), paroxetine (Paxil), escitalopram (Lexapro), and citalopram (Celexa). Prozac has become a household word. It was the first to be approved by the FDA, in 1987.[3] SSRIs increase the level of serotonin in the synapse, at least initially, and ultimately contribute to regaining a sense of well-being. Side effects may include sexual dysfunction, nausea, headache, insomnia, and upset stomach. These drugs *inhibit* or block the reuptake. Do not take the dietary supplement St. John's Wort if you are on SSRIs as they may interact.[4]

SEROTONIN NOREPINEPHRINE REUPTAKE INHIBITORS (SNRIs)

These drugs target both serotonin and norepinephrine neurotransmitter systems in the brain. The group includes duloxetine (Cymbalta), venlafaxine (Effexor), and mirtazapine (Remeron). Side effects may include dry mouth, headache, sedation, nausea, and tremors.

NOREPINEPHRINE-DOPAMINE REUPTAKE INHIBITORS

The most widely used drug in this class is bupropion (Wellbutrin, Zyban), and it blocks the brain's reuptake of dopamine and norepinephrine. Bupropion was the first nonnicotine drug approved by the FDA for treating cigarette addiction. It can lead to seizures at high doses, agitation, anxiety, and trouble sleeping. It is not usually associated with sexual problems or weight gain (in fact, some people lose weight on it).

TRICYCLIC ANTIDEPRESSANTS

This was the first group to come on the market and they are still prescribed today. They include amitriptyline (Elavil), clomipramine (Anafranil), imipramine (Tofranil), desipramine (Norpramin), and nortiptyline (Pamelor). Tricyclics work by increasing the amount of neurotransmitters in the synapse, again by blocking their reuptake pumps. Common side effects include weight gain, constipation, dry mouth, lowered blood pressure, and dizziness. They are anticholinergic drugs.

COMBINED REUPTAKE INHIBITORS AND RECEPTOR BLOCKERS

These antidepressants have sedative properties. Drugs include trazodone (Desyrel) and nefazodone (Serzone). Reported side effects are dry mouth, sleepiness, dizziness, a fall in blood pressure upon standing, upset stomach, and occasionally painful, sustained erection in men.

STIMULANTS FOR DYSTHYMIA OR LOW MOOD

Sometimes doctors prescribe methylphenidate (Ritalin) or dextroamphetamine (Dexedrine) to treat a mood disorder called dysthymia that is less severe, but more chronic, than major depression. They work more quickly than antidepressants to pep you up, increasing energy and facilitating attention and concentration. Common side effects include nervousness, insomnia, constipation, headache, and changes in heart rate.

MONOAMINE OXIDASE INHIBITORS (MAOIs)

MAOIs are effective, but physicians do not prescribe them often because they have potentially serious side effects from drug-drug and drug-food interactions.

Anxiety Medications

As with depression, those who are battling or have battled cancer sometimes report feelings of anxiousness that may also respond to medications. Benzodiazepines (BZs) are one class of drugs used in the treatment of anxiety and insomnia. Unlike antidepressants, they work almost immediately. The drugs include lorazepam (Ativan), alprazolam (Xanax), diazepam (Valium), clonazepam (Klonopin), chlordiazepoxide (Librium) and triazolam (Halcion). Some people do become dependent upon BZs, but the drugs are generally safe when used for a short time or intermittently as needed. Short-term side effects include psychomotor retardation, that is a slowing of reaction time, drowsiness, poor concentration and memory, and mental confusion (so they may not be the best class of drug to take if you already suffer from those types of symptoms, except just before bed, in treatment of occasional insomnia). It is not a good idea to take BZs—even a low amount—with alcohol, as the two together can be a fatal combination. Women who are pregnant or nursing should also avoid BZs. If taken with opiates, such as morphine, codeine, oxycodone, or a number of other painkillers in this class, ask your doctor about adjusting your dose because the drugs can be more potent taken together than individually.

Other medications include the anti-anxiety agent buspirone (Buspar), which tends to produce fewer adverse short-term effects on central nervous system function such as memory problems or sedation. As with the BZs, buspirone should be avoided by pregnant or nursing women. Some of the drugs in the antidepressant category are also used to combat certain kinds of anxiety, such as fears related to socializing, panic disorder, and obsessive rumination.

Dietary Mood Elevators

If you're averse to taking medication, there are other ways to increase neurotransmitters in the brain without the use of synthetic drugs, which can be worth a try.

SEROTONIN

Found in animal and plant protein, tryptophan is an essential amino acid that increases levels of serotonin in the brain, so it produces a calming effect. We also know that a depletion of tryptophan will depress your spirit. In fact, scientists in the Netherlands were among the first to show that you can induce negative moods biologically by restricting the level of tryptophan in people's diets.[5]

Tryptophan may also boost melatonin, a hormone secreted by a small endocrine gland in the brain that is associated with inducing sleep. Tryptophan is plentiful in chickpeas, beans, poultry, cheese, salmon, sesame and sunflower seeds, milk, eggs, and bananas, among other foods.

ACETYLCHOLINE

The brain makes acetylcholine from choline, an essential nutrient that is found in fat molecules called phospholipids. The most common form is phosphatidylcholine, also in the food supplement lecithin (derived from egg yolks or soy). According to the Linus Pauling Institute Micronutrient Information Center, adequate intake levels of choline for adults are 550 milligrams per day for men and 425 milligrams per day for women.[6] You will find relatively rich sources of choline in food portions such as 3 ounces of pan-fried beef liver (355 mg), 1 cup of toasted wheat germ (172 mg), 1 large egg (126 mg), or 2 cups of chopped cooked broccoli (126 mg).

NOREPINEPHRINE AND DOPAMINE

The natural synthetic pathway of these neurotransmitters begins with phenylalanine, an essential amino acid that converts into tyrosine. In turn, tyrosine boosts levels of dopamine and norepinephrine. Phenylalanine is found in protein-dense foods such as eggs, soy, nuts, and animal products. Phenylalanine and tyrosine are also available as nutritional supplements, and are sometimes used in that form for the stimulatory, antidepressing effects mediated by the catecholamine neurotransmitters. When used in this way, they should be taken with vitamin C and B complex supplements (which can be found combined into one formulation, often marketed as "anti-stress" vitamins) to promote their absorption.

For anyone suffering from depression and/or anxiety, it's important to recognize the symptoms and get treatment because no one should have to live with emotional pain. And if you happen to also struggle with cloudy thinking, then taking those steps may lead to another end: recovery of your cognitive abilities so that you are once again the person you were, before cancer and chemotherapy.

CHAPTER 14

Sleeping Through Insomnia

The National Cancer Institute estimates that 12 percent to 25 percent of the general population and about 45 percent of people with cancer experience sleep disturbances.[1] Worry and depression are the most common contributors to insomnia in otherwise healthy people. Pain and some cancer treatments, especially regimens containing mind-revving steroids can also interfere with sleep. And if you talk to people who are experiencing hot flashes and night sweats from early onset menopause, they will tell you a thing or two about insomnia. Lack of sleep quite literally messes with your head. Taken to the extreme, sleep disturbances can cause disorientation, depression, even delusional or psychotic behavior.

We see much higher levels of depression, stress, and anxiety in people with chronic sleep problems. These symptoms are particularly pernicious in that respect because they can entrap you in vicious cycles. Stress and anxieties interfere with sleep, as anyone who has lain awake in bed for hours worried about how they're going to deal with the next day's tasks (which may have also been the previous day's challenges) knows all too well. Feelings of guilt have the same effect. And major depression—which can be induced by chronic stress and can cause feelings of excessive guilt and anxious thoughts and behaviors—is also associated with sleep disturbance.

To make matters worse, sleepiness clouds judgment and other aspects of cognitive performance. In a study comparing sleep deprivation versus alcohol intoxication, scientists in Australia and New Zealand found that people who drive after staying up for seventeen to nineteen hours performed worse on tests of response speeds and accuracy measures than those who had a blood alcohol concentration of 0.05 percent.[2] Performance deteriorated even further after longer periods without sleep, becoming as bad as that found in someone having a 0.1 percent blood alcohol concentration (equivalent to four rapidly consumed alcoholic drinks by an average adult male). Just to put that into driving safety perspective, in Sweden you are considered legally impaired while driving if your blood alcohol content is greater than or equal to 0.02 percent. (In Australia, Belgium, and Greece that number is 0.05 percent; in most of Canada, the United Kingdom, and the United States it is 0.08 percent.[3])

Why Do We Sleep?

This may be one of the great evolutionary mysteries in all of science, though sleep is as important to our survival as nourishment, and as cognitively essential as the ability to form memories and make sense of the world.

Mammals sleep for at least two reasons. One is to become physically restored. For this purpose, we actually do not need to sleep per se, but only to hold still for several hours so that the connections between nerves and muscles can be retuned. We generally get this rest lying down because standing would require continued exertion of our muscles.

We also sleep to restore brain function. Just being awake requires the brain to use a substantial amount of energy—an average of about 25 watts (which, from a standard incandescent light bulb, would yield an amount of light equivalent to the output of sixteen dinner candles [200 lumens] . . . and from an energy-efficient, twisty compact fluorescent bulb would provide more than 120 candles worth of light). The brain generally uses only glucose for fuel—a simple sugar that is a main energy source for all cells in the body. So we need a protracted sleep period to refuel our brains.

The Best Advice: Sleep on It

The most important thing that happens during sleep is what goes on in our brains. When we sleep, we consolidate information. We hook up all that we have experienced since the last night's sleep to all that we previously knew, even from years prior. We integrate the day's memories into long-term storage. That lets us infer what the new material means in the bigger context of our lives.

In one fascinating study from Harvard Medical School, fifty-six college students initially learned five pairs of information.[4] What the students were not told was that each pair contained an embedded hierarchy of patterns. The researchers wanted to see which group could best make judgments about how the information related to each other in the hierarchy.

The students comprised three groups and each tested at different timepoints: twenty minutes later, twelve hours later with half having slept, and twenty-four hours later after all had slept. The students who were tested twenty minutes after learning the material showed no ability to infer the hierarchy. The twelve-hour and twenty-four-hour groups demonstrated that the time delay enhanced their ability to make the inferences, but those who had slept demonstrated the biggest boost in relational memory, or in understanding the significance of the material.

Bedtime Cycles

There are five stages of human sleep, the last of which is REM—what all the other stages lead up to—characterized by rapid eye movements where our brains are active and we experience our usual type of dreams (as opposed to, for example, "night terrors"). REM is normally preceded by four stages of non-REM, involving increasingly deep sleep. We sleep in cycles of about ninety minutes after the initial cycle of sleep, which requires two to three hours to complete, and go through a total of four to five cycles during a typical good night's sleep. Most of our time is spent in non-REM during the first part of the night, while REM takes up an increasing portion of our time as we continue sleeping into the early morning hours. The five stages of sleep occur in a particular order:

> **Stage 1**—This is the transition between waking and sleeping where if someone abruptly woke you up and accused you of dozing, you might deny it because you do not yet feel asleep. But you sink into relaxation. Your breathing and brain activity slows. You may be there for about ten minutes.

> **Stage 2**—This is still a light sleep, but conscious awareness disappears. We spend about half of our time sleeping in this stage throughout the night.

Stages 3 and 4—We are in deep or slow wave sleep, so called because if you monitor the brain with EEG electrodes, you will see the electric waves in the brain slowing down as you move from stage to stage with four being the deepest sleep. This is where our brain gets its best chance of refueling since its own energy needs are lowest.

REM Sleep—It typically takes us a couple of hours to get into REM after initially falling asleep. The first cycle of REM may last only ten minutes, lengthening each time up to an hour. So we may wake in the midst of a long period of dreaming. It is in REM where we soak up the best cognitive part of sleep. REM has a lot to do with excitation or the firing of neuronal circuits as they connect new information to old. In fact, if you want to analyze a friend's dreams, you can often make sense of them if you know enough about that person's past and what he or she experienced the previous day.

A Good Nap

If you have time during the day, twenty- to thirty-minute "power naps" appear to help prevent information "burnout" or frustration, irritation, and poorer performance on mental tasks. In one study on napping sponsored by the National Institutes of Health, subjects performed four daily practice sessions of a visual task.[5] As fatigue set in, their scores dropped over the sessions. But for those who took a thirty-minute nap after session number two, their scores declined no further. Subjects who took a one-hour nap at that point actually boosted their performance in the third and fourth sessions.

But timing is important in napping. If you power nap too long, you run the risk of waking from slow-wave sleep (Stage 3 or 4). We have all been there: that groggy, sluggish, cranky feeling where you (and others around you) wish you had not napped at all. If you have the time and need for a two- to three-hour siesta, you can awaken even more rejuvenated, having had the opportunity to get all the way through the energetically restorative slow-wave sleep, as well as the mind-building REM sleep. But don't expect to fall asleep as early or as easily, or sleep as long, when nighttime comes around.

Strategies for Better Sleeping

Wake at the same time each morning.

Exercise daily—the best exercise is the kind that wears you out, leaving you feeling spent but mellow and relaxed. Aerobic walking or swimming is great for that. At the very least, do stretching exercises each day.

Do not drink alcohol before bed as a sedative or to dull emotional pain. Alcohol at bedtime will help you fall asleep, but as it wears off, you will lose the ability to stay asleep.

Cut out caffeine in the late afternoon and evening.

Develop a relaxing nighttime routine. The right time to get in your day's worth of exercising (see above) is not right before you're ready to go to bed!

Keep note paper and a pen near your bed. If you awake anxious in the night, write down what is worrying you. Tell yourself you will look at it in the morning and get back to sleep. What your brain does during REM will help you face—and possibly even solve—your problems the next day, much more effectively than lying awake ruminating about them throughout the night.

ABOUT SLEEPING PILLS

Sleeping pills are generally fine for occasional use, but most of them have been shown to be REM suppressive. So not only might you wake up groggy, but you might not get as much mind-building done in your sleep as you normally would. Sleeping medications can be addictive, leading to tolerance and dependence if you take them regularly. Over the long term, it is far better to find ways to fall sleep without them.

If you have been through cancer, or if you are dealing with it now, then you may be familiar with benzodiazepines, the same class of drugs often prescribed for anxiety and for agitated depressions. Two well-known drugs in this group are lorazepam (Ativan) and diazepam (Valium). Benzodiazepines work by slowing down the central nervous system, creating a sedative and hypnotic effect, and helping your muscles relax.

Another well-advertised agent is zolpidem, known by its trade name, Ambien. One of the problems with the original formulation of zolpidem is that the sedative effect wears off during the night, so some people wake early. A newer controlled-release formulation works longer, but it is more expensive and not yet available generically. If you ask your doctor to specify the drug by its brand name on your prescription and add, "DAW" (dispense as written), that will assure you are getting the original manufacturers' versions of drugs. Many insurers will provide increased reimbursement for the more expensive brand-name products. But you often must have health insurance with prescription medication coverage and give available generics a good-faith try. Your physician may also need to document that the generic drugs failed to provide adequate relief.

SPOTLIGHT ON MELATONIN

Melatonin is a hormone produced naturally in the body and by other living organisms such as algae. It is also sold as a dietary supplement to help with regulating the sleep-wake cycle. But melatonin may be good for more than getting to sleep on time. Researchers are now wondering if melatonin might help prevent and treat breast and other cancers. An interesting characteristic of the hormone is that it is intricately tied to our circadian rhythm, our twenty-four-hour biological clock. That is, our brains secrete melatonin at night but suppress it during the day. Should you wake at night and turn on a lamp, your brain's melatonin factory shuts down production. It resumes only after darkness reclaims the room.

In recent years, Eva S. Schernhammer, M.D., DrPH, an epidemiologist at Brigham and Women's Hospital in Boston, along with her colleagues have studied data nested within the Nurses' Health Study, a more than decade-long investigation looking at risk factors for major diseases among thousands of female registered nurses. They found that higher melatonin levels as measured in a woman's first morning urine sample are associated with a lower risk of breast cancer.[6] They also associated years of rotating night-shift work with an increased risk of breast cancer and colorectal cancer in women.[7]

So what does that mean for you? First, much more research needs to be done before doctors should routinely prescribe melatonin supplements for cancer prevention, although work in the field is indeed promising. But it is also a good idea to try to maintain a healthy sleep cycle.

Whether this is done by following lifestyle strategies for better sleeping or by occasionally taking sleep-inducing drugs, a good rest means a sharp mind.

CHAPTER 15

Fatigue, Inattention, and Poor Concentration

Anyone who has suffered from cancer-related fatigue will tell you that no matter how many hours you log sleeping at night or napping during the day, there just is no relief. Small daily tasks loom before you, daunting and insurmountable. Your world presses along, slow and heavy. You feel the drag behind your eyes. You just want to curl up, knees to chest, but life goes on. You are late for work. You are low on groceries. Appointments lurk on your calendar. Your family needs you. You marshal your energy and push yourself away from the couch.

Among cancer survivors, fatigue is often profound. In a study sponsored by the American Cancer Society of 752 patients from three states who had been diagnosed the previous year with one of the ten most common cancers, approximately two-thirds were concerned about fatigue and loss of strength.[1] In fact, that was their second greatest concern, ranking just after fear of recurrence.

Nonprescription Remedies

RETURNING TO NATURE

We all know that enjoying the great outdoors can be therapeutic. But when people hear it also may help restore attention, generally the response is, "Really? Looking at a bunch of trees can do that?"

But it seems that actively appreciating nature for a limited amount of time each week helps correct or improve "attentional fatigue" while undergoing treatment for cancer. Attentional fatigue is what happens when our ability to focus and concentrate drains away. We may get easily distracted and lose our train of thought. Most people just get frustrated or impatient with themselves over these lapses. But for people diagnosed with cancer, attentional fatigue can be more debilitating. It can interfere with taking in information and thinking through major decisions.

In one study, researchers looked at nature's effects on attention in a population of newly diagnosed, mostly early stage breast cancer patients before and after surgery.[2] They tested two groups. One was the "nature" group and included eighty-three women. The other was a control group of seventy-four women with similar diagnoses who did not participate in the nature exercises. Everyone took batteries of tests within three weeks after diagnosis. They had not yet had surgery or any treatment.

The nature group spent at least two hours each week experiencing nature in whatever way they liked. They could watch or listen to birds or other sounds of nature, gaze at a sunset, or admire the clouds, stroll in a scenic area or garden, or even sit by a window with a view of greenery. The control group logged their minutes, relaxing and/or in free-time activities.

Three weeks after surgery (lumpectomy or mastectomy), but before chemotherapy or radiation, each group took their second battery of tests. About thirty-six days had passed in between. Even the women who had mastectomies resumed their nature activities just days after surgery. They did what they could manage physically, whether it was watching snow fall at the window or having someone take them on scenic drives.

The women who had been exposed to a natural restorative environment showed significantly greater recovery or improvement in their capacity to direct attention compared to the control group. The study concluded that regular exposure to nature could give newly diagnosed cancer patients a head start in halting or counteracting attentional fatigue during the weeks and months after surgery.

Indeed, that was the case in following up on these women after the initial study. Patients were evaluated three more times over the course of about one year. The women in the intervention group maintained improvement in their attention. It did not seem to matter whether they had chemotherapy alone or with radiation treatments, or had radiation alone.

What apparently did matter was making sure that they interacted with the natural environment and that they avoided mental effort while doing so. The researchers incorporated the work of University of Michigan psychologist Stephen Kaplan and his attention restoration theory.[3] His theory relies on four properties. Try them yourself, and see if they help restore your attention.

Property No. 1: Being Away From Your Everyday Environment

"Away" could mean tending your garden. Interacting with nature, says the researchers, "helps an individual move away from tired cognitive brain structures that have become fatigued through overuse." A diagnosis of cancer is so stressful that focusing on it is almost more of a mental strain than we can bear. The effort costs us dearly. It literally tires us out, zapping our energy. It robs us of our ability to attend. It is "getting away," or changing scenery if you will, that restores us emotionally. But it is still possible to exert mental effort while you are away. That is self-defeating. So there must also be . . .

Property No. 2: Fascination

What engages us requires no mental exertion. What is more captivating than the copper blush of sunrise or sand crabs at low tide burrowing themselves beneath the ocean's edge? Our attention there would be involuntary—not directed. So "fascination" mentally restores us.

Property No. 3: Extent or Scope

You are away and fascinated by what you behold or touch or inhale or hear. But can you remain there for a reasonable time without getting bored? Do you feel safe there? If you feel safe and satisfied, then you will not need directed attention to function. So you have sufficient extent or scope.

Property No. 4: Compatibility

You have interacted with the environment in a way that is compatible with you. Gardening may not be your thing. You may prefer walking in the woods near your home or bird watching.

We asked lead author of the study Bernadine Cimprich why nature is such an important requirement to getting away to another mental space. Why not just flip on the TV and zone out into a near-vegetative state?

"The theory has an evolutionary perspective to it," she answered. "The human brain is wired to respond to the natural environment in a very spontaneous kind of way because we had to survive in that environment. So we have a natural attraction to green, to trees, to water, to wildlife, to flowers and plants, and to animals. And when they are in our environment, we pay attention to them using a different attentional system than would be used whenever one concentrates on a mental task."

In other words, natural restorative activities help you see the forest *and* the trees. Over time, they help you reflect, "clearing the head of unfinished thoughts and interactions, making sense of events, [while] confronting nagging or painful problems," says Cimprich. Overall, you benefit with rested attention and mental clarity. Both are important when dealing with cancer.

CAFFEINE

Caffeine is a different kind of nonprescription remedy. The stimulant occurs naturally in coffee, tea, cocoa, and in the leaves or fruit of plants such as the guarana or kola nut tree. Manufacturers add it to soft drinks and other products.

There are decades worth of research that show clear-cut benefits of caffeine. It sharpens cognitive function, improves accuracy and speed in performing tasks that require sustained attention and concentration, and promotes alertness and a sense of well-being. People with chronic dysthymia or mild depression often find that caffeine boosts their mood. Beware of caffeine if you have heart problems, though, as caffeine can exacerbate cardiac arrythmias. If you're pregnant, check with your doctor about caffeine use. Keep in mind there is more caffeine in brewed coffee than instant and more caffeine in instant coffee than tea. Here are some comparisons from the Center for Science in the Public Interest:[4]

Coffee: 8 oz brewed (133 mg) • 8 oz instant (93 mg) • 8 oz Decaffeinated (5 mg)

Tea: 8 oz Brewed (53 mg)

Soft drinks: 12 oz Jolt Cola (72 mg) • 12 oz Mountain Dew, regular or diet (54 mg) • 12 oz Diet Coke (47 mg) • 12 oz Pepsi (38 mg)

Energy drinks: 8.3 oz Red Bull (80 mg)

Chocolate: 1.45 oz Hershey's Special Dark Chocolate Bar (31 mg)

Over-the-counter drugs: 1 tablet No Doz (maximum strength) (200 mg) • 1 tablet Vivarin (200 mg) • 2 tablets Excedrin (extra strength) (130 mg)

AMERICAN GINSENG

Another naturally occurring plant product may also help. Debra Barton, Ph.D., is a registered nurse and a researcher at the North Central Cancer Treatment Group based at Mayo Clinic in Rochester, Minnesota. She and her team have recently completed a well-controlled pilot study of American ginseng. Theirs is the first to evaluate the effectiveness of Wisconsin-grown ginseng to treat cancer-related fatigue.

Herbalists refer to ginseng as an *adaptogen* because they believe it restores balance to the body and helps the body resist fatigue, stress, anxiety, and trauma. The two most common types of ginseng are Asian (*Panax ginseng*) and American (*Panax quinquefolius*). Asian ginseng is typically grown in China and Korea. American ginseng is native to eastern North America, but wild ginseng has been driven nearly to extinction there by aggressive harvesting. Today it is mostly cultivated in more Western parts of the United States (Minnesota and Wisconsin) and in Canada (British Columbia and Ontario), as well as in parts of China to where it has been transplanted.

The results of the American ginseng study were promising. About 175 people completed the randomized, placebo-controlled trial (more enrolled initially, but some dropped out). The researchers divided the participants into four groups, receiving 0, 750, 1,000, or 2,000 mg daily of American ginseng. Dr. Barton said no one complain of side effects.

After eight weeks, the group getting the 0 mg placebo and the group with the lowest dose of ginseng showed little improvement in fatigue. But approximately one-fourth of the subjects in the two groups receiving the larger doses reported improvements in overall energy and vitality and less interference with activities due to general fatigue. They also reported an improvement in overall mental, physical, spiritual, and emotional well-being.

Dr. Barton cautions people to be careful about grabbing ginseng supplements off supermarket shelves because not all ginseng is created equally. "For cancer survivors, there are issues with how it's processed," she says. "Some places manufacture ginseng root through a process called alcohol extraction. When you use that, the ginseng has been shown to have estrogenic properties. That can be very serious for people who need to stay away from estrogen."

The manufacturing process is rarely mentioned on the label, says Dr. Barton, who tells the story of walking into a vitamin store that is part of a well-known national chain and speaking to the manager: "I asked him, 'How do I know that this is what it says it is? How do I know that there's not contaminants in there? How do I know how it was manufactured?' He couldn't answer any of those questions."

Still, she understands that people are going to want to get the same ginseng that participants received in the pilot trial. They used plain ground root, produced for them under strict standards set by the Ginseng Board of Wisconsin. There was no extraction process used, although in the follow-up study, the researchers plan to use water extraction to increase the ginsenoside content or potency. Dr. Barton refers people to the Ginseng Board of Wisconsin Web site (www.ginsengboard.com) where there is a link to a summary of the pilot study along with contact information for obtaining the same formulation of ginseng.

"I can tell you that the dose we have proposed to study in the next trial is 1,500 milligrams, that is 1,000 milligrams in the morning and 500 milligrams no later than noon," she says. "There are some data suggesting that American ginseng could lower blood sugar, so people on antidiabetic medicines should not take this without their doctor's knowledge and oversight. Also because of that, we do recommend (in the study) that people take it after eating."[5]

Prescription Pharmaceuticals

You may be taking in scenes of nature a half hour each day and drinking a cup of coffee first thing in the morning and in the mid-afternoon (or perhaps you prefer several cups of tea). You may be also getting 1,500 mg of high-quality American ginseng each morning. And still, if you are having trouble mustering the energy and concentration to get through a simple magazine article (or this sentence!), you may want to talk to your doctor about prescription medications. None has as yet been specifically approved for this purpose, and none is without risk. But a number of drugs in the stimulant category have long been prescribed for combating fatigue and concentration/attention disorders due to noncancer-related causes.

One of the cheapest and best studied is methylphenidate (marketed as Ritalin, Concerta, Daytrana, Metadate, and Methylin). Most primary care physicians are familiar with methylphenidate and know what to watch out for as they have been prescribing it for decades to treat narcolepsy and attention deficit disorder. So, if you and your physician do decide that prescription stimulants are right for you, methylphenidate would probably be a good first choice. It would make sense to proceed to newer (and costlier) stimulants only if you do not respond well.

Two other stimulants that show promise specifically for this type of fatigue are modafinil and dexmethylphenidate (described in more detail below). The initial data are encouraging. But we have yet to see published results of large-scale definitive investigations that have tested these drugs with patients who suffer from cancer-related fatigue.

MODAFINIL (PROVIGIL)

The Food and Drug Administration approved modafinil in 1998 to treat excessive daytime sleepiness associated with narcolepsy and other sleep disorders. Sadna Kohli, Ph.D., MPH, at the University of Rochester, and colleagues wanted to see if the drug, which is marketed to "improve wakefulness," would help with persistent fatigue in patients who had been treated for cancer.

So in 2004, the researchers began enrolling breast cancer patients in a randomized clinical trial to test the drug. The women who participated (eighty-two enrolled/sixty-eight completed the trial) had all complained of fatigue as well as problems with memory and concentration. Each took 200 mg daily for four weeks. Half then continued for another four weeks. Those who completed all eight weeks on modafinil reported major improvements in levels of fatigue, as well as with concentration, memory, and learning. Specifically, they were able to recall numbers, words, and pictures more quickly than the control group.

Aside from a couple of complaints of headaches and one of nausea, side effects were minimal. Modafinil is in a class of drugs called eugeroics, which are designed to stimulate the brain only when needed, to avoid the jitteriness and highs and lows that you sometimes see with amphetamines and other stimulants. The effects of modafinil appear to last for about twelve hours.

Brenda's Story

"I felt a difference the first day I took the full dose," says Brenda Oathout, now fifty-eight and a participant in Dr. Sadna Kohli's original modafinil study. "It was absolutely incredible; I was myself again." Brenda describes her prior self as the kind of person you would go to if you wanted something done. She was an energy force, juggling corporate life as a busy executive, organizing parties, serving as secretary of her bowling league, and skipping around town with the grandkids on weekends.

But then came surgery, radiation, chemotherapy, and hormonal treatment for breast cancer and two and a half years of debilitating fatigue. "I couldn't do anything anymore," says Brenda. "I had absolutely no desire to even talk on the phone. I was tired; I couldn't think."

Brenda is a partner in a financial services firm in Rochester, New York. "I'm expected to perform at a certain level," she says. "I was having a lot of memory problems. I would go blank, totally blank."

The modafinil helped thaw the brain freeze, says Brenda, reporting that her cognitive test scores before and after the drug kicked in were like "day and night" and that her fatigue has completely lifted.

She continues on the drug today, obtaining it with a doctor's prescription but "off-label," meaning not for the drug's intended purpose as approved by the FDA. Since the FDA does not regulate the practice of medicine, licensed physicians can still prescribe the drug if it is

FATIGUE, INATTENTION, AND POOR CONCENTRATION

medically appropriate. Brenda's insurance will not cover the drug, though.

"I pay $742.48 per month," says Brenda, calculating her out-of-pocket cost to the exact penny. Will she pay for it for the rest of her life? "If I have to," she says.

DEXMETHYLPHENIDATE HYDROCHLORIDE OR D-MPH (FOCALIN)

A drug used for the treatment of attention deficit and hyperactivity disorder (ADHD) has also shown some promise in treating cancer patients diagnosed with chemotherapy-related fatigue and cognitive dysfunction. The drug is dexmethylphenidate hydrochloride or d-MPH (brand name Focalin). It is a specific form of methylphenidate (Ritalin) that is most often prescribed for ADHD. Like modafinil, it works by stimulating the central nervous system. In its extended-release formulation, Focalin XR, it can also be taken in once-daily doses.

"I heard an interesting comment while waiting to get scans done in Nashville yesterday. One of the ladies in the lobby said she did a "chemo brain check" in the morning while going through treatment. I asked her what that was, and she said she tried to remember something significant: her grandchildren's birthdays or her social security number. If she could not do those two things, she knew to

CONTINUES

153

be careful on those days and to be sure she didn't leave the stove on, forget to take her medications, etc."

—Richard, Nashville, Tennessee. Melanoma recurrence, stage 3, diagnosed in 2006 at age sixty-four. (Treatment: surgery. Chemo: cisplatin, vinblastine, dacarbazine and interferon.)

TABLE 15.1: Side-by-side drug comparison of Provigil (modafinil) and Focalin XR (dexmethylphenidate hydrochloride)

DRUG SPECIFICS	PROVIGIL®[1] (MODAFINIL)	FOCALIN XR®[2] (DEXMETHYLPHENIDATE HYDROCHLORIDE)
Dosage	Tablets: 100 and 200 mg strengths. Adults: initially 200 mg each a.m., may increase to 400 mg each a.m., if needed (begin with 100 mg each a.m. if have severe liver dysfunction). Not approved for use in children under sixteen years old.	Extended release capsules. May be swallowed whole, or beads may be sprinkled on applesauce and swallowed immediately; do not chew, crush, or cut beads. 5, 10, 15, 20 mg strengths. Adults: initially 10 mg each a.m., may increase to 20 mg each a.m. after 1 week, if needed.
Availability	Prescription only	Same
Category	Stimulant of the central nervous system	Same
Possible Side Effects	Nausea, headache, dizziness, insomnia, anxiety, nervousness or infection, and skin reactions that can become permanently disabling, disfiguring, and life-threatening.	Abdominal pain, nausea, loss of appetite, fever, insomnia, overstimulation, anxiety, weight loss, dizziness, increased blood pressure and heart rate, Tourette's syndrome, psychosis, seizures, blood disorders, rash, visual disturbances, and tics

[1] *http://www.fda.gov/cder/consumerinfo/druginfo/provigil.HTM*
[2] *http://www.fda.gov/cder/Offices/ODS/MG/dexmethylphenidateXRMG.pdf*

TABLE 15.1: (continued)

DRUG SPECIFICS	PROVIGIL®1 (MODAFINIL)	FOCALIN XR®2 (DEXMETHYLPHENIDATE HYDROCHLORIDE)
Precautions (not a comprehensive list)	Can interfere with birth control (pills, patches, shots, and implantable devices) so use alternate methods during the time you are on modafinil and for one month after stopping the drug. There may be potential risks to babies who are breastfed. Let your doctor know if you are pregnant or thinking of becoming pregnant, or if you have problems with blood pressure or your liver, or if you have a history of mental illness or a recent heart attack. If so, modafinil may not be safe for you. Modafinil may interact with other drugs, including clomipramine, cyclosporine, hormonal birth control agents, rifampin, desipramine, triazolam (Halcion), diazepam (Valium), warfarin (Coumadin), phenytoin (Dilantin), and alcohol.	Discontinue in the event of seizures or agitation. Do not take if you have high blood pressure, hyperthyroidism, recent heart attack, marked anxiety, glaucoma, tics, Tourette's syndrome in you or your family, psychosis, epilepsy, or substance abuse. Monitor blood pressure and complete blood counts, including differential and platelets. May interact with MAOIs taken within two weeks, anticonvulsants, anticoagulants, antidepressants, and other medicines that lower or raise blood pressure.

[1] *http://www.fda.gov/cder/consumerinfo/druginfo/provigil.HTM*
[2] *http://www.fda.gov/cder/Offices/ODS/MG/dexmethylphenidateXRMG.pdf*

CHAPTER 16

Fear, Stress, and Mindfulness

Even in times of normal health, chronic stress as well as fear and anxieties about a future that we feel helpless to control ultimately can lead to depression. In turn, depression can lead to a mental fog. So imagine how that stress—and fog—intensifies when you're dealing with cancer. You are suddenly faced with fears about your own mortality. And before you can even process those fears, you are thrust into making a flurry of treatment decisions that may range from distressing to horrific. What you think, what you decide, literally may affect whether you live or die. It is no wonder then that facing the consequences of those decisions and dealing with concerns about potential recurrence or spread of your cancer, can propel you into a downward spiral. Stress, fear, and anxiety can produce a debilitating drop in energy, mood, and cognition. All this further contributes to agitation, stress, and anxieties about how you will manage to accomplish even the most basic requirements of your day-to-day life.

The good news is, there are things you can do to break the momentum. For starters, just talking about it with someone you trust is a healing act—whether that is your oncologist or family doctor, a psychiatrist or counselor, a pastor or rabbi, an empathetic friend or spiritual guide, or members of a cancer support group such as the Wellness Community or Gilda's Club. It may also help to keep in mind that literally hundreds of thousands of people have been where you are now and have risen beyond it. More specific techniques and remedies will be found in the chapters that follow.

How Stress Affects Your Mind

Short-term stresses release a chemical cascade of events that begin in a part of your nervous system and rapidly affect your brain and every kind of muscle in your body. We know this stress reaction as fight-or-flight, a response that is so primitive and hardwired into our genetic makeup that from the beginning of human existence it has helped ensure our survival. This response is what helped your ancestors defeat or escape fierce jungle predators. When we perceive danger, our sympathetic (fight and flight) nervous system shoots out norepinephrine, and the medullary (central) part of our adrenal glands pumps epinephrine (also called adrenaline) into the bloodstream. The norepinephrine and epinephrine then cause our smooth muscles to open up the blood vessels that supply oxygen and fuel to our brain, as well as to the muscles of our arms, legs, chest wall, and heart. At the same time, our parasympathetic nervous system (which activates body processes appropriate to more relaxing circumstances, such as digesting a meal, or defecating) shuts down . . . which is why, when we are agitated and hurried, we may lose our appetite. As a result of all these fight and flight reactions, our pulse quickens. We breathe harder. Our pupils dilate. Our livers release more glucose into our blood to provide extra energy to our muscles and brain.

These kinds of short-term stresses are our physical and emotional tigers and have stayed with us through evolution. We release these stress chemicals when someone cuts us off on the highway and when our "Type A" personality kicks into overdrive. When the threat disappears, we can relax. Our brain calls off its "red alert." Our sympathetic nervous system slows. Our parasympathetic nervous system resumes its maintenance functions.

But there are also long-term stresses that may damage the brain and the immune system over time. This happens when our brains remain on "orange alert," when we feel helpless, perhaps when we have been ill and when worry and grief consume us. When that happens, we release another set of hormones, the best studied of which is called cortisol. We release this hormone from the cortical (outer shell portion) of our adrenal glands and pump it into our bloodstream.

We even know from blood and amniotic fluid samples of pregnant women who are stressed that high amounts of cortisol will affect the neuroendocrine systems of their developing fetuses.[1] Biologically, these babies will be more sensitive to stress.[2] This reaction is a striking example of something that can be inherited without being genetic (two distinct concepts that are often confused). Inherited means a trait is passed down from generation to generation. And a low-stress tolerance can be passed from mother to fetus without any direct gene involvement at all. Over the long term, cortisol suppresses our immune systems, and we become less able to fight off infections. Too much cortisol will also directly affect the brain . . . for example, cortisol can shrink cells in the hippocampus, a part of the brain that is necessary for forming and accessing memories.

Calming the Fight-or-Flight Response

As mentioned above, just as stress is associated with one set of physical reactions, relaxation is associated with another. The systems in our body affected by stress return to their normal state. If you feel chronically stressed or anxious or fearful, it is especially important that you use well-established methods to induce the relaxation response. There are a number of techniques available, as you will see. In Marlene's case, she had to first realize how deeply she was hurting.

Marlene's Story

The facilitator looked at the emaciated young woman, her bald head wrapped in a yellow bandana. "You can do this, I know you can. Look at what you've been through already," he said. It was true. Marlene had undergone surgery for a particularly aggressive form of cancer, endured chemotherapy, and soon faced weeks of radiation treatments.

But this was different. Here she was on a chilly morning, literally walking a plank, the tip of which hung over a mountain cliff high above the mist-capped evergreens of Malibu, California. Were she to fall, she would tumble hundreds of feet to her death. Marlene sobbed, scared out of her wits.

"The harness will hold you," he reassured her. "All you have to do is jump." Marlene wasn't so sure. The harness looked secure enough. It was hooked to a thick cable that was anchored to a three-ton SUV. But what if the rope snapped? What if her harness came loose?

She looked at the twenty other women sitting to the side on boulders near tumbleweeds in the brush, all waiting their turns, all cancer

CONTINUES

survivors. They had been instructed to communicate encouragement with their eyes, but not to speak. Most cried with her.

"Now," said the facilitator, "tell me what you fear."

At first, Marlene said nothing. She stood doubled over, holding her stomach. Finally, she whispered, "I don't want to die."

"Again, say it again louder," he commanded.

She straightened up. Her face was soaked and puffy. "I don't want to die!"

"Now walk to the end of the plank and let go," he said. "Let go of your fear!"

Inch by inch, Marlene trembled her way to the tip of the plank . . . and jumped. But instead of cascading to her death, the cable held her safely in the air. She stretched out her arms like an eagle suspended in flight. Then the women heard a new emotion. This was something raw and split open. This was fury born from the deepest of insults. "God damn you, cancer!" she screamed. "You will not get me! I *will* see my kids grow up! You stay the f-k away!"

The facilitator pulled her up, unhooked her from the harness, and folded her into his arms. "You did it, Marlene. You did it."

Thanks to the dedicated work of two healthcare workers, Marlene is one of more than nine hundred cancer survivors who have attended these weekend retreats in the Malibu Mountains. In 1994, Nancy Raymon, RN, an oncology nurse specialist, and Donna Farris, LCSW, a clinical social worker, founded the nonprofit organization Healing Odyssey (www.healingodyssey.org) to help people move quickly and powerfully through illness and live fully, without paralyzing fear.

There are few organizations like Healing Odyssey. Women of all ages, who have experienced any type of cancer, whether in active treatment or a survivor for years, find themselves literally sheltered at a refuge with others who know what they have gone through. They attend workshops and outdoor activities focused on mental, social, spiritual, and physical healing. By the time they head home Sunday afternoon, most are spent from the intense program, but they leave with coping strategies that many say—even years later—are what helped them take charge of their recovery.

Of course, you don't have to travel to the mountains of Malibu. There are other strategies you can use, no matter where you are, to break free of those effects of stress coursing along your neurons and through your bloodstream. Look through the following suggestions, pick ones that suit your personal orientation and situation, and see what works best for you.

SPIRITUAL MAILBOX

One exercise that some people find useful involves writing a letter to a spiritual higher power. You might try it. Find a quiet place, perhaps outside under a shade tree. Begin with "Dear ____," and fill in whomever or whatever that spiritual source is for you, whether it is specifically religious ("Lord") or more secular ("Mother Earth"). In the letter, you vent or share your darkest fears and anxieties about your illness or about a potential recurrence or about how cancer will affect your family and your future. You re-read the letter, and then you write back, responding to yourself as if *you* are the higher power.

As Raymon explains it, the return letter is often the most cathartic part of the experience. She encourages people to "just let go and let it happen," a kind of role-playing stream of consciousness. But if you can imagine your higher power answering you, especially in a moment of crisis, you gain a deeper understanding of yourself and what you truly believe, she says. "People will tell me that the response was so loving that it generated a feeling of hope and strength," says Raymon. "For a lot of people this is the first time they have really connected with their spirituality in a way that's meaningful."

The exercise actually originated with Raymon's own spiritual advisor, Rabbi Elie Spitz of Congregation B'nai Israel in Tustin, California, who calls it "cosmic empathy." The technique is rooted in Jewish folk practice where for at least the past two hundred years, Jews praying at the Western Wall of the Old City of Jerusalem have stuck prayers written on scraps of paper (in Yiddish called *kvittels*) in between the crevices of the Wall. "It's supposed to be a direct line, a spirtual mailbox," she says.

You don't have to stop with the two letters. Raymon advises an ongoing conversation. You can use this tool in the middle of the night when you are anxious and alone or when you don't want to wake your spouse or partner, or when it is too late to call your best friend.

COGNITIVE DISTORTIONS

Raymon and Farris work hard in these sessions to show how fear leads to thinking in absolutes. Here are some actual examples from cancer patients:

- This new pain means my cancer is back and that is catastrophic.
- There is a 75 percent cure rate for my cancer. I am probably in the 25 percent group.
- I will always feel fatigued.
- No one will look after my children if something happens to me.

- My doctor didn't call me back with the test results. It must be bad news.
- People tell me I look great, but they just feel sorry for me.

This is about obsessing on what is irrational, says Farris, when generally the facts play out differently. The following shows how she illustrates that point in the group setting. Try it on your own.

On a grid with columns, Farris writes down one woman's fear across the top: "Now that I am ill, my husband will leave me." In the first column, Farris has the woman quantify that fear on a scale of one to ten to show its importance. The woman says it is an "eight."

For the second column, Farris asks how often she experiences that fear. The woman answers, "about twice a week." Farris writes that down.

For the third column, Farris asks, What does that fear *do* to you? Then she writes the woman's answers: "I can't sleep, I overeat, I get really bitchy at my husband for no reason. I have low self-esteem."

Farris brings out a giant red stop sign and holds it up to make a visual point: Recognize and stop your irrational behavior. She tells her to reframe her fear based on what she knows to be true, and the woman says, "I can see I am jumping to conclusions. My husband is at my side at all of my doctor appointments. He wouldn't do that if he didn't really love me and care about me."

Farris reminds the group that not all fear is bad. Sometimes it motivates you in positive ways, such as being more vigilant about diet and exercise or seeing the doctor when something seems wrong.

ACTION FEARS

Action fears are fears where you have to actually *do* something to make them go away. "You can't just sit there and write about them," she says. Examples might be starting to date again, clearing up your finances, or buying a new home.

SIMPLE BEHAVIOR MODIFICATION TECHNIQUES

When nurse practitioner Sherry Goldman, R.N., C.N.P., sees patients as director of Patient Services at the Revlon/UCLA Breast Center, they often pour out their hearts to her, and she knows how hard it is for them to avoid dwelling on negative thoughts. A couple of quick tricks she recommends are:

- Wear a loose-fitting rubber band around your wrist. The moment you begin to obsess, lightly snap the rubber band. The quick sting will attach a consequence to your negative thinking and hopefully—literally—snap you out of it.
- Allow yourself a certain amount of time each day to feel sad or worried if that is what you need to do to process what is going on in your life. But limit it to just once per day and for a short period, say five to ten minutes. Then move on, perhaps by picturing yourself in a place you love to visit and allowing your mind to go there.

EXERCISE

Physical exercise increases cerebral blood flow and promotes the growth of brain cells. We know that when laboratory animals exercise regularly, they create new neurons in the hippocampus (an area of the brain essential for learning and memory). Inactive animals do not. Research also shows that physically active people have lowered risk for Alzheimer's disease. Exercise is also probably the single best natural stress reducer. So try to get in at least twenty to thirty minutes of aerobic exercise at least three to four times per week. By *aerobic*, we're not talking about excessive, but aim to exercise with at least enough vigor to achieve a sustained elevation of your pulse. For most, the resting pulse is sixty to one hundred beats per minute. Try to increase it to at least 120, though not higher than the pulse rate that is safe for you. For people of average cardiopulmonary fitness, this is often estimated by the following formula:

220 – your age x .85
(For example, for a sixty-year-old, 85 percent
of 160 equals 136)

But if you have not been exercising regularly, or if you have problems with your heart or lungs, consult with your doctor about safe levels. The endorphins that exercise releases serve as natural painkillers and also elevate our moods as in the "runner's high." If you are currently in treatment, then vigorous exercise may not be an option at the moment. Still, try to get out a few times during the week for a walk in the neighborhood and for some fresh air. The physical stimulation will not only help clear your head but will help combat persistent fatigue.

Often when people are stressed, they think, "I don't have time to exercise." But that view is based upon (erroneously) looking at time devoted to exercise as a one-way expenditure, showing up only on the "loss" side of your balance sheet. Actually, it adds considerably to the "revenue" side. For example, people who exercise will sleep better. Better sleep means less is needed because you are getting more high-quality sleep in a shorter amount of time. And even four to five hours of high-quality sleep is more restorative than eight to ten hours of tossing and turning, taking longer to fall asleep, and waking up frequently through the night with fragmented periods of REM. So exercise leads to better sleep. That leads to shorter sleep and to more time and energy during the day. You will find you are handling the day's activities with greater efficiency, more creativity, and in better spirits.

ACUPUNCTURE

Practitioners of this ancient Chinese form of medicine treat patients by inserting thin needles through the skin at specific points on the body to correct energy imbalances and boost the immune system. Acupuncture has been used effectively to treat chemotherapy-caused nausea, chronic headaches, backaches, menstrual cramps, and arthritis. Needling at the acupuncture points triggers the release of neurotransmitters and other chemicals that dull painful sensations and promote healing.

In just the last few years, Western scientists have begun to look at acupuncture as an effective treatment for cognitive dysfunction.[3] Functional magnetic resonance imaging (fMRI) has shown that acupuncture activates specific regions of the central nervous system that are responsible for high-level cognitive roles. In studies of dementia, it appears that acupuncture may prompt blood vessels to dilate, increasing oxygen supply to the brain. In studies of stroke patients, it may stimulate brain plasticity to aid recovery. There is even some evidence suggesting that acupuncture may be as effective as medications to treat depression and anxiety. Acupuncture is considered extremely safe with very few reports of any serious side effects. Knowing all that, there seems to be no downside to trying acupuncture. There also seems to be every reason for doctors to support their patients' decisions to do so.

YOGA

Yoga is an ancient mind-body discipline, originally practiced in India some five thousand years ago. It still draws many of us to its teachings of tranquility and physical and spiritual balance. In the last few decades, scientists have taken a closer look at yoga. They found that in addition to the sense of well-being that cancer survivors experience from its lessons of directing conscious thought, yoga also helps improve their fatigue, quality of sleep, depression, and cancer-related distress.[4]

Patients with a range of diagnoses, including lymphoma, breast, and prostate cancers, participated in these studies. Most practiced gentle poses and stretches from a variety of yoga disciplines. Some included meditation and breathing exercises that can help calm fears about cancer treatment or recurrence.

One pilot study at UCLA looked at the effect of Iyengar yoga on persistent cancer-related fatigue, a style chosen for its restorative poses and because even people with limited flexibility can participate. Iyengar yoga instructors generally go through rigorous training and testing before they can be certified, and they must pass an even higher standard of testing to teach therapeutic classes. So they can adapt the poses for people who need to be careful about aggravating lymphedema, a condition where lymph fluid accumulates in arms, hands or legs after lymphatic vessels or nodes have been removed.

Eleven women attended these classes twice each week for twelve weeks and kept a diary of how they were feeling. They reported significant increases in energy and continued to take classes on their own, even when the study ended. Because of the preliminary results, the researchers are now conducting the first randomized, controlled trial of Iyengar yoga and its effects on fatigue in breast cancer survivors. They will also collect data on how it impacts depression, pain, sleep, and pro-inflammatory cytokine activity. As discussed in more detail in Chapter 21, cytokines are a family of inflammatory molecules that are generally produced by white blood cells, or sometimes cancer cells. Pro-inflammatory cytokines seem to be elevated in some survivors who are fatigued and in others with cognitive dysfunction.

In a different study on sleep at M.D. Anderson Cancer Center in Houston, yoga also helped with insomnia.[5] About twenty lymphoma patients participated in seven weeks of Tibetan yoga classes while patients in a control group were offered no special intervention. As with Iyengar yoga, the Tibetan yoga used in the study was low impact. The instructors incorporated visual imagery, regulated breathing, and mindfulness techniques. The yoga group reported falling asleep more quickly than the control group, sleeping longer, and relying less on sleeping medications.

MEDITATION MAY REPAIR DAMAGED BRAINS

There are various forms of meditation. One is Transcendental Meditation, the technique that originated in India where with eyes closed you repeat a mantra or phrase to quiet the mind. Another is mindfulness, a Buddhist practice focusing on respiration or the flow of breath. The idea is that if you are mindful or aware of the sensations you are experiencing in the moment, you will learn to balance and accept your thoughts and feelings without judgment. A third type is Tai Chi, an ancient Chinese martial art involving deliberate and flowing movements to help balance the body's vital energy. Qigong is also a Chinese therapeutic art with deep breathing and Tai Chi–style movements.

Not only does meditation heighten attention and quiet the fight-or-flight response, but there is compelling evidence that it may actually help repair a damaged brain and strengthen the immune system.

Richard J. Davidson, Ph.D., is a neuroscientist at the University of Wisconsin-Madison and a pioneer in the field of East-West medicine. He is known for a remarkable collaboration with the Dalai Lama. The spiritual leader sent eight of his monks to the university so that Davidson could map their brains while they meditated. These particular monks were highly accomplished. Each had from fifteen to forty years of traditional Tibetan meditation experience.

Davidson also recruited a control group of ten students who had never meditated and gave one week of training to each. He and his team hooked up both groups to electrical sensors to measure their gamma brain waves and instructed the participants to meditate on the concept of unconditional loving-kindness and compassion. The researchers found powerful electrical activity in the monks with far more synchrony of gamma waves in their brains compared to the students.[6] That is, different parts of their brains experienced gamma waves at the same time. Presumably, this showed that meditation changed their brains' electrical patterns. The monks with the most years of meditation experience had the most synchronous gamma wave activity. Using fMRI in other studies involving the monks, Davidson has been able to show that increased blood flow occurs in the same area of the brain responsible for positive thoughts and emotions.

In a separate study, Sara Lazar, Ph.D., and her colleagues at Massachusetts General Hospital discovered that brain regions associated with sensory processing and attention were thicker in the subjects who meditated, documenting for the first time this link between brain structure and meditation. Further, they found that cortical thickness was especially pronounced in older subjects who meditated. Generally, as we age, the cortex thins in this area associated with emotional and cognitive processing.[7]

What does all of this research tell us? That not only do our brains continue to develop past adolescence, but they have a changeable quality called *neuroplasticity* at all stages of adulthood. This *plasticity* continues throughout our lives as our brains change in response to our social and emotional experiences, contrary to what neuroscientists originally believed possible.

Even if we are predisposed to depression or fear or anxiety, we can actually rework the function and structure of our brains to perceive life with a higher and happier level of awareness.

If you have not tried meditation before, you might start with the following exercise designed to induce the relaxation response. This meditation was created by Malcolm Schultz, J.D., M.F.T., clinical supervisor at The Wellness Community-West Los Angeles, in California. He has been leading similar meditations there for the last ten years.

Meditation for Reducing Stress and Enhancing Mental Clarity

This meditation may be practiced for any length of time, from five to thirty minutes per session and up to one hour if you are experienced. There is no limit on the number of sessions per day. Even five-minute meditations can seem like a long time for the new practitioner, so start with what is comfortable for you.

1. Sit in a chair with both feet flat on the floor. Keep your **spine reasonably straight**, neither rigid nor slumped. You may also sit cross-legged or, if necessary, lie flat on your back.

2. Place your **hands on thighs, palms up, tips of thumbs and forefingers touching, and fingers slightly separated.**

3. **Close** your **eyes**. If this is uncomfortable, leave them open. Form an **intention** to use the next ____ minutes to relax and to meditate. Choose an amount of time you think you can accomplish.

4. **Focus** your attention on your **breathing** without trying to change it in any way.

5. While continuing to focus on your breathing, **substitute a silent repetition for your thought process**. You may repeat silently "one" on the inhale and "two" on the exhale. Or you may use any uplifting word, short prayer, or mantra.

6. After your silent repetition is well established, imagine that a beautiful, crystal-clear **light** is **filling** your **mind** with great awareness.

7. Whenever you notice that your attention is involved with random thoughts, gently **refocus** on the breathing and the silent repetition.

8. Continue this process for the intended period of time.

Courtesy, Malcolm Schultz, J.D., M.F.T., clinical supervisor, The Wellness Community-West Los Angeles, CA.

CHAPTER 17

Brain Food

Minding Your Fats

We've all heard a lot about fat, how it is bad for us, bad for our hearts, our arteries, our brains. But that's not necessarily true. *Some* fat in our diets is healthful. Certain fats are even essential to well-being. They energize us, satisfy hunger, and aid in maintaining cell membranes and steroid hormone production. We also know that the brain regulates almost all systems of the body to some extent. So fat can either promote good brain health—or impair it. What's important is to separate out the good fats from the bad.

FATS THAT ARE BAD FOR BRAINS AND OTHER LIVING THINGS

Saturated Fats and Trans Fats

The molecules in saturated fats and trans fats pack together closely so they are solid not only while refrigerated, but also at room temperature. Saturated fats increase the amount of cholesterol your body makes. Both types of fat can cause atherosclerosis, or clogging of the arteries. That in turn can increase the risk of heart attack and stroke (which is essentially a "brain attack," or the death of brain cells caused by poor blood flow—and not enough oxygen—to the brain).

Cheese, whole milk, butter, lard, and other fatty animal products are loaded with saturated fat. Plant-based saturated fats include coconut oil, palm oil, and palm kernel oil.

Trans fats are found mostly in baked goods, snack foods such as popcorn and potato chips, salad dressings, margarine, shortening, prepared mixes, and fried foods. A few cities like New York and Philadelphia have banned the use of

Instead of dressing, try mashing a ripe avocado into your salad (or knead it in with your fingers to get it everywhere). Add a few shakes of pepper and coarse sea salt or a few drops of Bragg Liquid Aminos for seasoning. Squeeze in a bit of lemon.

trans fats in restaurants, and California passed a similar law to phase them out from restaurants and bakeries.[1] Food companies are scrambling to find menu alternatives to their trans-fat-laden piecrusts, cakes, donuts, breads, and crackers. But still, these artery cloggers are everywhere, in some fast-food restaurants and probably on the ingredient list of at least some of your packaged or frozen foods at home.

Here are two things you can do to look out for your brain, your heart, and the rest of you:

- Check the ingredient list. The FDA now requires that manufacturers disclose trans fats on labels only if the food contains more than 0.5 grams of trans fat.[2] So, even if the package boasts "No Trans Fats," you may still find the words "partially hydrogenated vegetable oil" (and sometimes "shortening") in the ingredients list. That will tell you that the food contains some trans fats.

• When you purchase bakery items at a restaurant, ask if the establishment uses vegetable oil. If they do, ask if it is partially hydrogenated. If so, let them know that kind of oil is unhealthful. Ask if they can prepare your food with olive oil or canola oil instead. Customer satisfaction is a powerful motivator to influence change.

In contrast, you don't need to avoid most other types of fats unless you are counting calories. And we especially encourage consuming one particular kind of fatty acid, as you will see below.

THE BATTLE OF THE OMEGAS

If you're having problems with your thinking, then you'll want to know about omega-3 and omega-6 polyunsaturated fatty acids (assigned an "omega" number based on their chemical makeup). Our bodies do not manufacture omega-3 or omega-6 polyunsaturated fatty acids. So we must metabolize them from food. These fats are essential to our diet. Without them we would not be able to function normally. The devil is in how much omega-6 we consume. Too much might cause disease-promoting inflammation over the long term. In the case of omega-3 fats, though, well-controlled research shows they are among the good guys. Omega-3 fatty acids are crucial to brain development both before and after birth, and to maintaining optimal brain function and vision. Docosahexanoic acid (DHA), a type of omega-3, is the most abundant fatty acid in our brains.

The richest source of DHA is oily cold-water fish. Species such as salmon, mackerel, herring, trout, anchovies, and sardines provide us with it by feeding on phytoplankton—microscopic plants that contain DHA and another form of omega-3 called eicosapentaenoic acid (EPA). Oily fish are also high in vitamin D, a nutrient that researchers believe may play a significant role in reducing the risk of diabetes, cancer, and heart disease. DHA and EPA are also present in algae, egg yolks, and some other foods as well.

Seafood Sources of Omega-3

Here are some sources of DHA and EPA (in milligrams) found in 6 ounces of cooked seafood.

TABLE 17.1: Sources of Omega-3 Fatty Acids in Seafood

6-OZ. PORTIONS (COOKED UNLESS NOTED)	(MG)	6-OZ. PORTIONS (COOKED UNLESS NOTED)	(MG)
Herring, Atlantic, Kippered	3,895	Halibut, Greenland	2,097
Herring, Pacific	3,739	Trout, rainbow, wild	1,999
Salmon, Atlantic, farmed	3,844	Salmon, coho, wild	1,895
Anchovy, European, canned in oil	3,524	Swordfish	1,798
Sablefish	3,247	Bluefish	1,680
Salmon, chinook	3,142	Bass, striped	1,677
Whitefish, mixed species	3,142	Smelt, rainbow	1,619
Sardine, Pacific, canned in tomato sauce	2,776	Tilefish	1,539
Salmon, sockeye, canned	2,598	Mussel, blue	1,398
Tuna, fresh, bluefin	2,559	Wolffish, Atlantic	1,378
Herring, Atlantic, pickled	2,363	Carp	1,355
Salmon, coho, farmed	2,305	Pompano, Florida	1,238
Salmon, pink	2,266	Pollock, Atlantic	922
Mackerel, Atlantic	2,238	Whiting, mixed species	903
Salmon, sockeye	2,198	Sturgeon, mixed species	844
Trout, rainbow, farmed	2,102	Crab, blue	842

CONTINUES

TABLE 17.1: (continued)

6-OZ. PORTIONS (COOKED UNLESS NOTED)	(MG)	6-OZ. PORTIONS (COOKED UNLESS NOTED)	(MG)
Oyster, Eastern, canned	810	Tuna, yellowfin, fresh	500
Rockfish, Pacific, mixed spices	791	Clam, mixed species, canned, drained	497
Salmon, chinook, smoked lox	765	Cod, Pacific	475
Ocean perch, Atlantic	760	Tuna, light, canned in water	463
Crab, Alaska king	726	Lingcod	447
Pike, walleye	708	Catfish, channel, farmed	441
Mackerel, king	682	Sheepshead	323
Catfish, channel, wild	566	Tilapia	306
Mullet, striped	558	Pike, Northern	279
Shrimp, mixed species	556	Cod, Atlantic	270
Snapper, mixed species	546	Gefiltefish, commercial, sweet recipe	204
Octopus	534	Lobster, Northern	143

Source: U.S. Department of Agriculture, Agricultural Research Service. 2007 USDA National Nutrient Database for Standard Reference, Release 20. Nutrient Data Laboratory http://www.ars.usda.gov/nutrientdata.

Plant Sources of Omega-3

To get omega-3 from plants, humans must first convert alpha-linolenic acid to the biologically active EPA and DHA. Experts disagree on how much, if any, we actually absorb. Those who study fatty acids say it takes about ten grams of alpha-linolenic acid to yield one gram of EPA and DHA.[3] So plant sources of omega-3 are not easy to come by. Many foods contain both omega-3 and omega-6 fatty acids.

Still, you will find the highest sources of alpha-linolenic acid in flaxseeds, canola oil, and walnuts. And even though flaxseed oil contains a lot more alpha-linolenic acid than the seeds, flaxseeds contain high amounts of healthy soluble fiber. There are also more lignans in the seeds, which are phytochemicals that help boost the immune system. Try ground flaxseeds mixed into a morning fruit or protein shake, or sprinkled on a salad.

Omega-3 fatty acids have anti-inflammatory and antioxidant properties, and multiple studies are underway testing them as anticancer agents. There is also some evidence that omega-3 fatty acids may play a role in decreasing risk of dementia and cognitive decline and in improving learning abilities and mood.

At UCLA, colleagues at the Alzheimer's Disease Preclinical Research Lab have been studying fatty acids and other nutrients for years, looking for doorways to potential cures for Alzheimer's disease. In one phase of research, they fed mice a diet rich in DHA and found that the fatty acid protected against protein loss in the brain synapses and prevented cognitive deficits.[4] They noted 40 to 50 percent fewer

TABLE 17.2: Plant Sources of Omega-3 and Omega-6 Fatty Acids

OMEGA -3	OMEGA-6
Flaxseed	Corn oil
Flaxseed oil	Soybean oil
Canola oil	Safflower oil
English walnuts	Sesame oil
	Peanut oil
	Primrose oil
	Borage oil
	Grapeseed oil
	Cottonseed oil

Source: U.S. Department of Agriculture, Agricultural Research Service. 2007 USDA National Nutrient Database for Standard Reference, Release 20. Nutrient Data Laboratory http://www. ars.usda.gov/nutrientdata

amyloid plaques in the brain, deposits associated with Alzheimer's disease. The team also found that, conversely, the mice that were fed a DHA-depleted diet suffered from cognitive deficits and a severe loss of synapse proteins in the brain.

In another study—this one involving people—scientists at the University of Siena in Italy tested the cognitive and physiological effects of omega-3 on thirty-three volunteers.[5] The participants consumed a total of eight 500 mg capsules of fish oil before meals each day (altogether containing 1,600 mg of EPA, 800 mg of DHA, and 400 mg of other types of omega-3 fatty acids daily) for thirty-five days. A control group received placebo capsules (containing only olive oil) for thirty-five days. All of the subjects went through psychological and cognitive testing on day one and day thirty-five of the experiment. By the end of the trial, the subjects on the omega-3 supplements demonstrated increased vigor and reduced depression, anger, and anxiety compared to the control group. They also showed improved attention in tasks involving complex processing.

Omega-3 also appears to boost anti-inflammatory properties and balance our immune systems. And a deficiency of omega-3 fatty acids may lead to a wide variety of neurological problems, including depression.

Omega-3 fatty acid is good for the heart, and we need good heart health to support the function of the brain as well as all of our other organs. Several studies show that omega-3 lowers both the "bad" kind of blood cholesterol (LDL) and triglycerides, a type of fat found in the bloodstream that is associated with diabetes and atherosclerosis (commonly referred to as "hardening of the arteries"). Atherosclerosis can lead to stroke and heart disease. Poorly circulating blood or blocked arteries also affect our brain's ability to work properly. So omega-3 fatty acids help promote healthy mental processing.

Questions About Farmed Salmon

Some experts in the field of cancer prevention and nutrition recommend avoiding farm-raised salmon, even though it contains high amounts of omega-3 fatty acids. They are concerned about the antiparasitic drugs that producers may be feeding these fish and worry about the buildup of chemicals in salmon from polluted waters. One reason is in 2004, scientists from Indiana University and from Cornell University tested seven hundred farmed and wild salmon fillets sold in markets in sixteen large cities throughout North America and Europe and discovered that farmed salmon had significantly higher concentrations of PCBs, dioxins, and other environmental contaminants than their wild counterparts.[6]

In general, large predatory fish tend to store the highest levels of contaminants. Tilefish from the Gulf of Mexico (also called golden bass or golden snapper), shark, swordfish, and king mackerel contain higher levels of brain-toxic mercury. See the list on page 180 for data from the U.S. Environmental Protection Agency that shows mercury levels in seafood. You will notice that salmon in general is low in mercury concentrations, although as the scientists pointed out, chances are farmed salmon is loaded with PCBs. And while wild salmon may actually provide a lower amount of omega-3 fatty acids than farmed salmon, the omega-3 content still ranks among the highest per ounce of all foods commonly consumed in a Western diet.

FISH OIL SUPPLEMENTS

Typical Dose: 400 mg/daily of DHA/EPA omega-3 fatty acids
Some people prefer to get their omega-3 fatty acids from supplements, but they worry about toxins in the fish oil as well, which is a reasonable concern. The Food and Drug Administration doesn't regulate supplements with the same scrutiny as drugs. The best we can

TABLE 17.3: Mercury Concentrations in Seafood
(In parts per million)

(SEAFOOD)	(PPM)	(SEAFOOD)	(PPM)
Tilefish (Gulf of Mexico)	1.45	Squid	0.07
Shark	0.99	Trout (freshwater)	0.07
Swordfish	0.98	Croaker (Atlantic)	0.07
King Mackerel (Gulf of Mexico)	0.73	Whitefish	0.07
Orange Roughy	0.55	Crab (Blue, King, Snow)	0.06
Marlin	0.49	Butterfish	0.06
Grouper	0.47	Scallop	0.05
Tuna (fresh)	0.38	Mullet	0.05
Bass, Chilean	0.39	Pollock	0.04
Tuna (canned albacore)	0.35	Catfish	0.04
Lobster (Northern/American)	0.31	Herring	0.04
Halibut	0.25	Anchovies	0.04
Bass, Saltwater, Black, Striped	0.22	Haddock (Atlantic)	0.03
Snapper	0.19	Sardine	0.02
Monkfish	0.18	Tilapia	0.01
Carp	0.14	Oyster	0.01
Perch (freshwater)	0.14	Salmon (fresh)	0.01
Tilefish (Atlantic)	0.14	Salmon (canned)	None detected
Skate	0.13	Shrimp	None detected
Cod	0.10	Clam	None detected
Lobster (Spiny)	0.09	Perch (ocean)	None detected
		Whiting	None detected

Source: U.S. Dept. of Health and Human Services; Environmental Protection Agency, Feb. 2006.

do is to rely on independent reviews from companies like Consumer Lab.com and Consumer Reports that test products for quality and safety. ConsumerLab.com reviewed forty-four brands of omega-3 fatty acid (EPA and DHA) supplements from fish and marine oils and found that none had detectable mercury or unsafe PCB levels. All but two were fresh.

If fish oil supplements make you burp or you continue to taste fish flavor afterward, there may be a reason: over time, fish oil can turn rancid. If your bottle of capsules seems to lose its freshness before you have finished it, buy smaller bottles, or keep your large bottles tightly capped and in the refrigerator.

Omega-6

Like omega-3, omega-6 is an essential polyunsaturated fatty acid that the body cannot manufacture on its own, and we must consume it to survive. Both fats produce eicosanoids—powerful chemical messengers. In the case of omega-3s, these messengers signal the body to boost the immune system and fight inflammation. But the story is different for omega-6s. As we metabolize omega-6 fatty acids, chemical messengers work in reverse. They promote inflammation, which at times can be a good thing. When we are sick or injured we want pro-inflammatory eicosanoids to initiate the healing process. The problem comes when our ratio of omega-3 to omega-6 fatty acids is out of whack. Too much omega-6 causes chronic inflammation. That can contribute to heart disease, allergies, and cancer. Most experts advise at least a one-to-four ratio of omega-3 to omega-6 for a healthful diet.

You will find omega-6 fats in fried foods, mayonnaise, cookies, cakes, chips, crackers, cereals, seeds and nuts and their refined oils (such as soybean, safflower, sunflower, cottonseed, and corn oil),

Instead of traditional mayonnaise, try vegan brands made with expeller-pressed canola oil. Instead of margarine, shortening, or butter, try soy- or canola-oil based substitutes.

grains, egg yolks, and in corn or grain-fed beef and poultry (the breast meat in chicken and turkey has less omega-6 because it is lower in fat).

Lessons From Early Humans

Piecing together data from fossils, ethnobiologists know that at one time in our evolutionary history, our ancestors consumed roughly a one-to-one ratio of these two fats. These hunter-gatherers basically ate two food groups: wild plants, and meat and fish. Dairy products did not exist in the Paleolithic diet prior to the domestication of animals some ten thousand years ago. Of course, the same is true for breads and cereals and other grain products. We began cultivating grains only some ten thousand to fifteen thousand years ago.[7]

Our ancestors' diet of fruits, roots, legumes, and nuts has helped anthropologists understand that omega-3 fatty acids were concentrated in the green leaves of plants (and in some seeds and nuts), while omega-6 fatty acids were concentrated in seeds also—and then later, grains. The deer they hunted had foraged on tall grasses and ferns. So the meat was leaner and contained omega-3. But today we domesticate cattle and lamb and pigs and chicken and feed them corn and other grains, and find them at supermarkets with fat full of omega-6.

Experts estimate that we now consume about fifteen times more omega-6 than omega-3 fats in our diets! That is not healthful. The bottom line is we need to cut out the junk. If you eat meat, look for grass-fed or avoid the animal fat. If you eat seafood, try to consume two servings of fatty fish each week. If you eat eggs, enjoy them. The whites are pure protein and fat free. And even though the yolks do contain omega-6 fats, cholesterol, and some saturated fat (look for omega-3-enriched eggs instead), they also contain a significant source of choline, zinc, phosphorus, and vitamins A and D.[8]

Finally, consider using olive oil or canola oil as your main oils for cooking and adding to salads or other foods. Consume more fruits and vegetables. And focus on foods that contain omega-3 fatty acids to balance out the omega-6 inflammatory molecules.

Brain-Friendly Antioxidants

We hear a lot about antioxidants; the term is everywhere in the promotion of bodybuilding and skincare products. So what are they? An antioxidant is a molecule that neutralizes "free radicals," which are oxygen molecules that have split and become unstable, wreaking havoc on your body and your brain.

CLEANING UP FREE RADICALS

The process works like this: Imagine that our bodies are like charcoal-fired barbecues. Just as coals give off heat, we burn or oxidize fuel, too, so that we can produce adenosine triphosphate (ATP), the energy molecule of cells. ATP is created in structures of cells called mitochondria. This process is not completely efficient and leaves behind free radicals. Like soot from the barbecue that gets on our hands, it spreads to everything else we touch at the picnic, from the spatula to the plate to the shirt on the guy who bumps into us.

So when we eat poorly, become stressed, breathe in cigarette smoke, absorb UV rays, or exercise too hard, we create unstable oxygen molecules or a kind of "soot" in our bodies. These free radicals steal electrons from other molecules, which then become new free radicals—a kind of chain reaction that leads to the creation of still more free radicals. Left unchecked, free radicals can damage the membranes that surround and protect all our cells, including in brain tissue, and they can even alter the structure of our DNA molecules, causing mutations passed on to the next generation of cells. They can contribute to neurological problems, early aging, and cancer.

We produce free radicals every single day. They're part of living, and we do have natural protectors floating around. Specialized enzymes in our white blood cells, vitamins C and E, and other dietary antioxidants (free radical "scavengers"), are examples. With insufficient defenses, some radicals get away and cause cellular damage.

COLORFUL FOODS FOR A GOOD MIND

Many plants produce natural compounds that shield against their own free radical generators. When we consume these plants, their antioxidant qualities protect us as well. Some of our best defenders are as near as our next meal—beta-carotene, lycopene, vitamin E, selenium, and vitamin C.

Beta-Carotene

Our bodies convert beta-carotene to vitamin A (retinal). This antioxidant enters our cell membranes and takes hits from free radicals, leaving cells intact. We get beta-carotene from yellow and orange vegetables such as carrots, sweet potatoes, cantaloupe melon, pumpkin, and mango. Generally, the more intense the color, the more the beta-carotene. We also find beta-carotene in kale, chard, parsley, and other dark green vegetables, their pigment masked by the color of chlorophyll. In fact, dark green leafy vegetables are also great sources of folic acid and B vitamins that may help with depression and memory.

Lycopene

Also in the carotenoid family, lycopene is beta-carotene's chemical cousin. Its red pigment is found in tomato, ketchup and spaghetti sauce, pink grapefruit, and watermelon. We absorb carotenoids best with fat. So chop, puree, and cook these foods with a little olive oil or canola oil.[9]

Vitamin E

Vitamin E (alpha-tocopherol) has been the subject of several cancer prevention and immune function studies because of its ability to neutralize free radicals, but results have been mixed. If you use diet to boost vitamin E, it is important to balance how much you consume of some of its richest sources since many are high-fat foods. Avocado, olive oil, canola oil, almonds, and hazelnuts are examples.

Selenium

Selenium is an essential trace mineral that works in tandem with vitamin E to combat oxidative stress. You will find both vitamin E and selenium in barley, brown rice, broccoli, Brussels sprouts, garbanzo beans, pumpkin, and pinto beans.[10]

Vitamin C (ascorbic acid)

Unlike the fat-soluble carotenoids and vitamin E, which watch over cell membranes (also full of fat), water-soluble vitamin C is like the U.S. Coast Guard, navigating through our waterways and protecting the bloodstream and the inner areas of our cells. Citrus fruits such as oranges and grapefruit are well-known sources of vitamin C as are sweet red peppers, strawberries, tomato, and broccoli.

PHYTOCHEMICALS

Phytochemicals are plant chemicals or the molecules that are responsible for the deep colors and aromas of edible plants. We see their presence in the color of blueberries, red cabbage, and red grapes, in chlorophyll-bursting bunches of parsley, and in the curcumin that brings us the yellow spice turmeric of Indian curries. We see it in the cocoa beans that produce dark chocolate and the mood-lifting chemical phenylethylamine. We see it in the herb rosemary that neuroscientists believe may shield the brain from stroke and neurodegeneration.[11] They also show up in the organic compounds resveratrol found in the grapes that produce red wine, in the isoflavones of soybeans, in the catechols in green tea, and in the indoles and isothiocyanates of broccoli. We smell their biological activity in garlic, scallions, and ginger.

We're constantly learning more about these plants' cancer-fighting, antioxidant, and anti-inflammatory properties, and there is evidence that phytochemicals may help protect brain cells as well.

So heap four or five colors onto your plate, and help yourself to some dark chocolate for dessert.

NO SURE BETS ON SUPPLEMENTS

Some people believe that dietary supplements are the answer to protecting our cells from free radical damage. It does make sense to take a daily multivitamin, but rigorously collected scientific data on most dietary supplements are virtually nonexistent. So you won't find any recommendations here to mega-dose. Our bodies are very efficient at handling small insults, but when we take large quantities of supplements, we may overwhelm our defenses. We risk adverse effects along with what is potentially good. What we do know—although often promising—is largely based upon unsystematically obtained data. With that caveat, here is what we presently presume to be true about a few supplements.

Vitamin D

There is considerable evidence that vitamin D is a potent regulator of the immune system and promotes normal cell growth. D is best known as the "sunshine vitamin" and has been used for decades to cure childhood rickets. In its active form, this fat-soluble vitamin changes to the steroid hormone calcitriol, which helps maintain blood calcium levels. Some evidence suggests that D decreases the risk of many common cancers (especially breast, ovarian, colon, and prostate), type-2 diabetes, autoimmune diseases, and high blood pressure.[12]

Most people, though, are deficient in vitamin D. Michael Holick, M.D., Ph.D., director of the Vitamin D, Skin and Bone Research Laboratory at Boston University Medical Center and the author of the book *The UV Advantage*, considers vitamin D deficiency "an unrecognized epidemic in both children and adults throughout the world."[13]

We're not assimilating enough from the vitamin D found in fortified foods, egg yolks, salmon, sardines, and other fatty fish. And although we manufacture vitamin D in our skin from exposure to sunlight, sunscreens and our justified fear of skin cancers keep us in the shade.

Dr. Holick says that just a few minutes of sun—five to fifteen minutes tops—a few days each week without sunscreen—will safely provide adequate levels of vitamin D (exposing arms and legs, or hands, arms, and face). In the absence of soaking up sunshine, he recommends vitamin D supplements added to a vitamin D–enriched diet so that we take in 1,000 international units daily of cholecalciferol (the chemical name for a form of vitamin D). Many brands of multivitamins already contain 400 units of vitamin D, and chances are your neighborhood pharmacy carries vitamin D supplements in 1,000 international unit formulations of cholecalciferol.

But don't take *too* much vitamin D. More than 2,000 units daily for six months can raise blood-calcium concentrations to toxic levels. So unless your doctor tells you otherwise, keep the supplement dose to about half that. Or you could hold your nose and gulp down a tablespoon of cod liver oil. With 1,360 units of vitamin D (and lots of brain-healthy omega-3 fatty acids!), it's more than enough to jump-start your day.[14]

Vitamin B_{12}

Vitamin B_{12} deficiency is a cause of *reversible* dementia. So ask your doctor to check your serum B_{12} level if you have memory problems. If it is lower than normal, then B_{12} supplements taken orally or through a shot could make a huge difference in your cognitive world. The B_{12} vitamin is not available in plants, so vegans especially need to make sure they get adequate amounts. Try to get at least six micrograms per day either through fortified foods or by taking supplements. Some people like the sublingual form that dissolves under the tongue for easier absorption. You will also find good amounts of B_{12} in animals and fish, and shellfish is especially high. Just 3 ounces of steamed clams will give you 84 micrograms of vitamin B_{12}.[15]

Coenzyme Q_{10}

Coenzyme Q_{10} is an important antioxidant that mops up free radicals generated during normal metabolism. But it appears to be a whole lot more than that. Every cell in our body makes coenzyme Q_{10}. It is a central component of the system that allows for ATP production, the energy source for all of our cells to stay alive and function. As we age, we lose the ability to produce coenzyme Q_{10}. That is a problem for the heart because it's the most oxygen-consuming organ in the body and has a huge number of mitochondria, the main energy source of our cells. The brain is loaded with mitochondria as well, and if those cells start dying, then we can develop neurodegenerative diseases.

There have been good studies showing the immune boosting effects of CoQ_{10}. And here is something you may want to know if you are undergoing treatment for cancer and are receiving the drug doxorubicin or daunorubicin. Clinical studies suggest that taking CoQ_{10} may not only enhance the anticancer effects of these agents, but it may prevent anthracycline-induced cardiotoxicity or the heart damage associated with these drugs.[16]

Other than reports of gastrointestinal symptoms, oral supplementation of CoQ_{10} in doses as high as 1,200 mg/day tested for up to sixteen months appears safe.[17] A typical dose, though, is 100 to 300 milligrams daily with food.[18]

There are some precautions. For example, do not take CoQ_{10} along with warfarin (Coumadin) without checking with your doctor as CoQ_{10} may decrease the drug's effectiveness.[19]

Ginkgo Biloba

A number of small trials have demonstrated that ginkgo biloba is a powerful antioxidant. But the science remains mixed on whether it helps memory and other cognitive abilities by improving blood flow to the brain. The big question is, does ginkgo protect against dementia? At least among those aged seventy-five or older, it appears not.

In the most rigorous clinical trial on ginkgo completed to date, more than three thousand elderly volunteers from five U.S. academic medical centers participated in the Ginkgo Evaluation of Memory Study between 2000 and 2008. About half received twice-daily doses of 120 mg extract of ginkgo biloba. The other half took a placebo. The study was "double-blind," meaning neither the investigators nor the participants knew who was getting what. As reported in the *Journal of the American Medical Association* (2008), the scientists found that ginkgo biloba had no effect in reducing the incidence of dementia or Alzheimer's disease in their subjects. (In fact, the incidence of dementia increased slightly among those taking ginkgo, and there were twice as many hemorrhagic strokes in that group as compared with the placebo group—sixteen versus eight).[20]

As a general precaution, ginkgo biloba may increase the risk of excessive bleeding, especially for people with blood circulation disorders and for those taking ibuprofen, aspirin, or other anti-coagulants.

Summing up all of this, even intuitively we know that good nutrition is not just about the body. What we consume has a direct relationship to our cognitive well-being. Omega-3 fats are linked to good brain (and heart) health; appear to protect against neurodegenerative diseases; and may help with mood, learning, and memory. Certain supplements and edible plants may be just as powerful. When we nourish the brain, we feed the mind.

CHAPTER 18

Some Tips for (Re)Organizing Your Day-to-Day Life

For some people, post-chemo brain lifts on its own or lessens over time. Others continue to suffer cognitive effects many years after treatment. Either way, here are some strategies to help you deal with it:

Stay present. Consciously tell yourself to focus, whether it is on a conversation or following the plot of a movie.

Prioritize. For most people with chemo brain, multitasking is impossible. Just the idea of having to accomplish two things at once can paralyze you into doing nothing at all. List your tasks in order of priority. Concentrate on one at a time. Tune out everything else.

Develop routines. Prepare for tomorrow the night before: Lay out your clothes, review your calendar at the end or beginning of the day (or both), exercise each day at the same time, and take medications routinely as well (use a pillbox with day-of-the-week labels).

Rehearse. You have a meeting or an appointment coming up, and you must be "on your game." Visualize the room or the people you will be seeing and literally practice what you will say. Watch yourself in a mirror if that helps.

Use word associations and rhyming. Susie "money bags" Gold; 8823 Cayne Street: He is eighty-eight and walks with twenty-three canes.

"Ever since I got lost in the shopping mall garage and couldn't find my car, I always write down the level number and color code, etc., on the back of my parking ticket. And I always place parking tickets in the same section of my purse so I know where to find them. For extra measure, I'll play a word game. If I'm parked on B1, for example, I'll make up a cue like: Be one with the universe."

—"M," breast cancer diagnosed in 2005 at age fifty-two.(Treatment: lumpectomy, radiation. Chemo: docetaxel, carboplatin. Targeted therapy: trastuzumab [Herceptin].)

Cue the senses. Partner people and places with their scents, sounds, tastes, textures, or unusual characteristics. Did he have a birthmark on his chin? Did the office building smell like old cheese? Connecting people and places with sensory cues helps with recall.

Break numbers into chunks. It is far easier to remember a phone number if you divide it into sections, such as 989 and 4423.

Ban scratch paper from your desk. People with post-chemo brain do not need little pieces of paper (especially sticky notes) and scribbles on the backs of envelopes all over their workspace. That will just make you nuts. Follow this cardinal rule: Use one solitary notebook for jotting down notes so that everything is in one central place. Even if the items in the notebook are disorganized, at least you know they are in there someplace. (It helps to date the pages as you use them.) This frees your desk—and your mind—from clutter.

Rely on day planners (or a paper calendar that is too bulky or large to misplace). Write down appointments immediately.

Use electronic calendars/organizers. The calendar feature on computer programs such as Microsoft Outlook will alert you in advance of appointments.

Post a checklist by the front door. "Remember keys, wallet, lunch, kids."

Post a list of frequently dialed phone numbers. Keep this near the phone you use most.

Label cell phones and landlines with their respective numbers. Have you ever tried to give someone your cell phone number while talking on it only to realize that you need to hang up first to find it on the phone's index function? If so, then this tip is for you.

Everything in its place. Keys, glasses, lists, organizers, anything that is important to you needs its own home so that you can always find it.

Simplify Your Life

Robert J. Ferguson, Ph.D., is a clinical psychologist at the Department of Rehabilitation Medicine, Eastern Maine Medical Center in Bangor, Maine, and an adjunct assistant professor of psychiatry at Dartmouth Medical School. He developed Memory and Attention Adaptation Training (MAAT) to help cancer survivors deal with cognitive decline after chemotherapy. Here are two of his more general tips.

Pick a time to go over your day planner or calendar. Most people eat breakfast or at least drink a cup of coffee in the morning. That routine is ingrained. So pair that behavior with your new routine to review your day's schedule.

Limit the amount of time devoted to e-mails. Check your e-mail from, say, 8 to 8:30 in the morning, and then you're done. An e-mail is, well, mail. "I don't run to my mailbox three times a day waiting to open up my letters," says Ferguson. "It is not intended to be instant messaging where you are available to be disrupted 24/7." After his half an hour is up, Ferguson sets the automatic reply on his e-mail function to say, "I may not respond to e-mails promptly due to volume. For any urgent matter, please call. . . . " He responds the next day, or the next.

Timers. Have a timer ring before the kitchen fills with black, stinky smoke because you have forgotten about the soup boiling on the stove that evaporates to nothing, which sets off the smoke detector and scares the living daylights out of you. Place it within hearing range.

"Whenever I see my oncologist, I experience brain freeze. He talks to me, and all I hear is, 'blah, blah, blah.' Now, I either take a friend with me who will recap things or I'll tape the conversation and play it back later."
—"M"

Leave messages for yourself on your voicemail or answering machine. This is helpful for reminding yourself of appointments and things you need to do.

Work your mind. Take a foreign language or a biology class at your community college. An acting class will help you memorize lines because of context of scenes. Join a monthly book club but attend every other month so that you will have two months to read each selection (get the list of all upcoming books). Enroll in a dance or exercise class where you can work on remembering the steps. Work a crossword or Sudoku puzzle (start with easy ones). Try some of the computer memory games, such as Posit Science Brain Fitness Program (www.positscience.com), Mindfit Back on Track (www.e-mindfitness.com), and Happy Neuron (www.happy-neuron.com). The handheld electronic "Brain Games" is based on research by Gary Small, M.D., chief of the UCLA Memory and Aging Research Center and on his book, *The Longevity Bible: 8 Essential Strategies for Keeping Your Mind Sharp and Your Body Young.*

Don't underestimate the power of rest, meditation, and yoga. All of these help with clarity.

Gum Chewing May Help Working Memory

It has long been hypothesized that chewing activates various brain regions. But there have been very few studies that look at the relationship of chewing to cognitive performance. Well, in 2008 a group of Japanese scientists published their findings of what is believed to be the first study to use functional MRI (magnetic resonance imaging) to examine the brains of thirty-one volunteers while they chewed gum during a working memory task. The researchers found that chewing increased the signals in the prefrontal cortex and activated other brain regions, including the hippocampus, during the tasks. The concentration and accuracy levels of the subjects increased as well. As they reported, "These results suggest that gum chewing may accelerate or recover the process of working memory besides inducing an arousal effect by the chewing motion, consequently enhancing cognitive performance."[1]

Keep a sense of humor. Although there's nothing funny about post-chemo brain, it's always good to maintain perspective. Everyone has something going on, right?

Dawn

I know that my sense of humor has grown since my diagnosis. When I was told I had cancer, I chose to go through treatment with dignity (did I say that?), grace (I ain't graceful; I'll tell you that after lots of falls and broken bones), laughing (I do so much love to laugh), and brainless (I ain't the sharpest tool anymore, but I am fascinated daily by the "new" me). As a script editor prior to chemo, it would take me about four to five hours to do a really good page-one edit. Now it takes me three weeks because by the time I get to page five, I've forgotten what happened to whom, and I need to start again.

I do believe that laughter is essential to recovery. Here is one funny—and true—story that I would like to share: Day one. My mastectomies. I woke up to find myself surrounded by family and friends. And the flowers, oy vey, the flowers. Too many to number, and they were sucking the oxygen out of what would be my room for the next ten days.

One arrangement stood out from the others. It was a beautiful white orchid, surrounded by these little beautiful yellow flowers that I still can't name. So I watered those flowers and I talked to them and I cared for them as if they were my only cord to the real world. The orchid died in days, but alas the yellow flowers flourished. I even got to take them home. To my bedroom. A constant reminder of the love that surrounded me during the first part of my journey.

Eventually I put the flowers on a ledge and watered them, talked to them, and took the best care of them that I could. I was going to live, damn it, and so were those flowers. For one year, I watered and talked and watered and talked. One day, I decided the leaves needed a cleaning and dusting, and to my amazement I thought the pretty yellow flowers had grown. I slowly slipped the flowerpot into my hands, being ever so careful not to spill the water. I looked closer and couldn't believe my eyes. Could it be? Was it possible? The flowers

CONTINUES

197

were fake! I had been watering a fake flower arrangement for one year!

Now, even five years after my mastectomies, when I see real yellow flowers, I laugh . . . and I also know that I will live.

—Dawn. Breast cancer, diagnosed in 2002 at age forty-seven. (Treatment: bilateral mastectomies, radiation. Chemo: doxorubicin, docetaxel. Anti-hormonals: anastrozole.)

PART V

How to Reclaim Your Brain Chemistry

CHAPTER 19

Nine Daily Steps You Can Start Doing Today
(But Wait Until Tonight!)

> *"Do not let what you cannot do interfere with what you can do."*
>
> —John Wooden, the most winning basketball coach in NCAA history, leading UCLA to ten championship titles and four perfect 30-to-0 seasons; the first person to be inducted into the National Basketball Hall of Fame as both a player and coach; recipient of the U.S. Presidential Medal of Freedom; and named by ESPN as "Greatest Coach of the Twentieth Century."

When considering all of the information discussed in this book up to this point, you might be wondering how to apply it to your life in particular. How can you use the information here to improve your own brain chemistry? Finally, is that information something you can apply daily?

If you expect a sudden cure or a fourteen-day program that you try one time and then forget, do not read beyond this paragraph! You're not ready to take advantage of this information any more than someone who wants to be thinner, yet is not ready to commit to long-term changes in diet and exercise. Put this book away for a day, or several days, or a few weeks . . . and don't pick it up again unless and until you decide you will do what it takes to think and feel better. Making this commitment (and meaning it) for some people may be the hardest step . . . but for all people, it is the most important one. There are no "quick fixes" to restoring the mind. If they existed, headlines would scream them.

But if you're ready to commit to a daily program of cognitive re-habilitation, one aimed at helping you make steady progress repairing your damaged brain chemistry, then read on. Your nine-step program is about to begin. Steps 1 and 2 start *tonight*.

The good news is, once you have committed (and we can safely presume you have, otherwise you would have stopped reading two paragraphs ago), you will embark on a course virtually guaranteed to lead to thinking and feeling better. How do you know you'll get better? Because yours will be a program based entirely upon the most solid, well-controlled medical research that exists today.

Wisely and humorously, the editor-in-chief of the *American Journal of Medicine*, Dr. Joe Alpert, recently distilled the essence of what might otherwise be found by working your way through dozens of self-help books, poring over hundreds of pages of research papers, and surfing through thousands of Internet sites, down to a handful of guidelines for achieving "Health, Happiness, and Longevity."[1] Here they are in an even more condensed form:

Inherit good genes

Never smoke!

Exercise daily

Don't starve yourself

Eat foods that are healthy

Don't get fat

Drink alcohol in moderation

Get preventive health care

Cultivate family and friends

Develop a hobby

Avoid daily TV news

Don't let little things get to you

From this advice we have created a practical, straightforward, nine-step program for treating post-chemo brain syndrome. Note that none of Dr. Alpert's prescriptions for a healthy life involve taking this or that over-the-counter formulation, or "health supplement." No wonder. Wading through the incomplete, confusing, and often contradictory massive amounts of information (and infomercials, and/or misinformation) about these products is enough to make anyone's head spin. Here are two generalizations to keep in mind:

Don't waste your time and mental energy (especially, as both are likely already in alarmingly short supply while enduring post-chemo brain symptoms)—not to mention your money—on supplements of unproven value (exception: unless you really want to waste them).

Most supplements are of unproven value (and some may occasionally harm you).

The reason for the exception to the first generalization is if you really want to try something because you are convinced it will help (and will do more good than harm . . . and won't dent your wallet!), then it might actually be helpful: the "placebo effect" is very real (it can even be measured with certain types of brain scanners) and can be very powerful, at least for a period of time. Conversely, if you strongly believe a product will not help you, even if that item has proven value, an equally powerful antiplacebo effect can prevent that substance from working.

Regarding the second generalization, there are good reasons why the U.S. Food and Drug Administration (FDA) requires marketers and distributors of health supplements to label their products as "not intended to prevent, diagnose, or treat any disease." (Yet people buy them for that very purpose). Some of those supplements might benefit the health of certain individuals, but the FDA does not have sufficient data that is of adequate quality to prove these products do more good than harm for most of the people who take them for specific ailments.

Keeping all this in mind and pulling together many of the principles in *Your Brain After Chemo*, here is a **Nine-Step Program to Reclaim Your Brain Chemistry**:

Steps 1 and 2 to Start Tonight
STEP 1: FOCUS EVERY DAY ON (ONLY) THOSE THINGS YOU CAN INFLUENCE OR CONTROL

As Alpert quipped in his article, "Try to be born into a family with a history of longevity." Well, even if we inherit good genes, as he advised in his list, and even if grandpa lives to 102, there are just some things we can't guarantee. Until gene therapy techniques make their entry into more routine clinical practice, there will still be plenty of us who live with genes we don't want. And even if you're born as hearty genetically as grandpa, you can still walk out your front door and get hit by a Mack truck. So let's keep things in perspective.

The effects of all genes critically depend upon a complex interplay between what's happening inside your cells (according to the instructions encoded in your DNA sequences) and what's happening outside your cells (the environment). Genes never operate in a vacuum; they cannot predetermine what will happen to your brain chemistry, and they do not represent your neurobiological destiny ... only your neurobiological predispositions. What actually happens to your brain chemistry will depend on the environment in which you immerse your brain (and its genes). You had no control over the genes packaged in the embryo that led to developing your brain. But you certainly can control many aspects of your brain's environment and general functioning, as you will see in the remaining steps.

There are practical reasons to focus on those things you can control. Sources of chronic distress can lead to chronically elevated levels of stress hormones such as cortisol that suppress your immune system. In turn, you become more vulnerable to getting sick with infectious diseases or even with certain kinds of cancer. Ongoing fear and anxiety can contribute to a "learned-helplessness" mindset. That by itself can induce depression. And depression can further impair cognition.

Beyond that, worry constitutes a self-depleting waste of physical and mental energies. This is poignantly expressed by the American writer and journalist Charles Fulton Oursler: "We crucify ourselves between two thieves: regret for yesterday and fear of tomorrow." And American storyteller Mark Twain put it this way: "I have been through some terrible things in my life, some of which actually happened."

But taking on realistic challenges boosts your acute-stress system. You release neurotransmitters into your synapses that activate your brain, and you pump adrenaline into your bloodstream. That action gears up your brain and the rest of your body to rise to the task. And when your mind is moving forward, you are far less inclined to get stuck and dwell on those things you can't do much about. Meditation and other mind-body techniques (see Chapter 16) can also help. And serotonin-specific or serotonin-norepinephrine-based therapy with a reuptake inhibitor (SSRI or SNRI) is well demonstrated to diminish obsessive and ruminating thinking patterns that can impair day-to-day functioning.

STEP 2: SET YOUR BIOLOGICAL CLOCK TO THE RIGHT TIME, AND KEEP IT RUNNING REGULARLY

An improperly set biologic clock will prevent you from getting the right kind of sleep. You will not be able to think straight (see Chapter 14). Even if sleep was never an issue for you prior to getting cancer, your diagnosis and/or your treatments may have thrown off your internal rhythms in any of a number of ways.

The simplest thing you can do to set and maintain your brain's clock to the right time is to control the timing of the light and darkness that your brain sees. Outdoor cues can help. They give your brain access to seeing the light-dark cycle that nature provides us, and with which our brains evolved. Provided you don't work at night or have other constraints, go to bed with your curtains open and your window shades up. Waking to the morning's first light or earlier time-sets the brain. Try to wake up at nearly the same time every day, regardless of when you go to bed. So if you normally get seven hours of sleep, say from midnight to 7 a.m., and Saturday night you party and don't get to bed until 3 a.m., you'll be much better off in the long run (and quite possibly, even during that Sunday) if you get yourself up Sunday morning around 7. Sleeping in until 10 or 11 a.m. will accost your brain with jet lag, the same as if you had flown from Los Angeles to New York overnight.

Bright, artificial lighting is the second best strategy for keeping your clock on track and will provide similar benefits. In fact, cognition and mood can be improved by simply turning on bright fluorescent ceiling lights at the same time every day.[2]

Steps 3, 4, and 5 to Start Tomorrow Morning

STEP 3: EAT PLENTY OF FRUITS AND VEGETABLES, ESPECIALLY THOSE WITH DARK COLORS

Dark-colored fruits and vegetables not only serve as the best source of natural fiber, minerals, and vitamins—some of which are essential constituents of the enzymes that synthesize neurotransmitters—but they also provide antioxidants that bathe your brain cells and other cells. For every day that you don't get at least five portions of fruits and vegetables, take a multivitamin. Most brain-critical vitamins are water soluble, meaning you don't store them up for "rainy days" when you don't get enough. Rather you pee them out on the "sunny days" when you get more than you need.

STEP 4: KEEP IN MIND THE 60/60 RULE

The other thing you need *every* day (because our bodies can't store it) is protein. If you're an average-sized adult who consumes about 2,000 calories per day, get *at least* 60 grams of protein, and *no more than* 60 grams of total fat. If you have trouble remembering this, just keep in mind that dietary habits are not really about grabbing lunch or sitting down for dinner. They are about what affects the fluid surrounding our brains, *each hour of the day*—sixty seconds to the minute and sixty minutes to the hour!

Note that if you're, say, a six-foot six-inch, 230-pound inactive guy eating 3,000 calories per day to maintain your weight, your diet should probably include more like 90 grams of protein. Even average-sized adults engaged in moderate to intense physical activity should probably take in protein two to three times higher than the 60 grams per day. Also, the U.S. Food and Drug Administration recommends that no more than 20 grams of your fat intake comes from saturated fat. Make sure you also get at least 0.4 grams (400 mg) of DHA/EPA omega-3 fatty acids (see Chapter 17).

Just as importantly, especially in the context of post-chemo brain, we need the amino acids in protein for a lot of things other than bulking up our muscles. They help us deal with acute stress throughout the rest of the body. The neurotransmission in our brains and our hormonal signals depend on them. Serotonin, norepinephrine, dopamine, GABA, glutamate, and adrenaline are *all* just slightly modified amino acids. All enzymes in the brain that synthesize the neurotransmitters from amino acids are big proteins. So are the channels for the sodium, potassium, and calcium ions that keep the electricity flowing through our neuropathways. So is the hemoglobin that carries oxygen to the brain (and to all our other tissues). And so is the hormone insulin that allows most of the cells of the body to get the glucose fuel they need. The same is true for all the antibodies that defend us from foreign invasion that can lead to release of cytokines. Similarly, proteins and shorter amino acid chains (peptides) form the molecules that are in charge of everything from digesting food fuels to regulating the level of thyroid-hormone stimulation throughout the entire body. So remember that the 60 gram rule is the *minimum* recommendation for daily protein intake—and as long as we have reasonably healthy kidneys, it would be really hard for us to get *too much* protein (regardless of what certain diets tout).

The 60/60 rule also suggests an easy definition for "junk food." Since you are trying to get at least 60 grams of protein without going over 60 grams of fat each day, a junk food in this context is anything that contains more fat than protein. Both a one-ounce bowl of Total whole grain cereal and a one-ounce bar of Dove milk chocolate contain 2 grams of protein. But the cereal contains 0.50 grams of fat, and the chocolate bar has 9.33 grams of fat. That means to get your 60 grams of protein each day by eating foods like the cereal, you would pick up 15 grams of fat. To get that amount of protein from items like the milk chocolate bar, you would take in 280 grams of fat (unless it's the smoother European-style chocolate . . . then expect to consume 360 grams of fat with your 60 grams of protein).

Does this mean you should give up eating candy bars? Not at all—there are actually a lot of good things you can get from chocolate. Chocolate serves as a rich source of quick fuel, caffeine, and other related compounds that stimulate your mind. It contains the compound phenylethylamine that serves as a precursor to certain neurotransmitter substances. Phenylethylamine may be a natural mood elevator, promoting feelings of contentment. Chocolate, especially the dark variety, might even help protect your brain tissue from further oxidative damage with its antioxidant compounds. Plus its biggest selling point . . . instant gratification! But if you are going to eat the chocolate bar, make up for it with more lean protein and less junk food throughout the day. That practice will keep you on course with the 60/60 rule.

To keep the math simple, think of dividing the 60 grams into four equal portions that you could combine any way you want over the course of the day. Fifteen grams of protein is about the amount contained within each of the following:[3]

- each 2-ounce half-portion of chicken, turkey, fish, pork, or beef
- each medium slice of pepperoni pizza
- two 8-ounce glasses of milk
- two 3.5-ounce servings of tofu
- two plain bagels
- three medium eggs
- one 2-ounce portion of Swiss or cheddar cheese
- one 3-ounce portion of mixed nuts
- one cup of cooked beans (pinto, baked, refried, black, navy, and lentils)
- 58 apples (i.e., don't depend on fruits for daily protein!)*

*For the purposes of completing this daily list, each day (twenty-four-hour period) ends shortly after breakfast. So, if after breakfast you find that this meal, along with the preceding day's dinner, lunch, and snacks, did not include four to five servings of fruit and vegetables, take a multivitamin pill. If you're not sure it included at least 0.4 g (400 mg) of DHA/EPA omega-3 fatty acids, take an omega-3 capsule. If it didn't include 60 g protein, spoon down a cup of blueberry yogurt for dessert or grab a protein bar on your way out the door. Your brain will thank you for the afterthought. Note also that the above two steps (3 and 4) are not intended to represent comprehensive guidelines for good health. For example, little attention is paid to dietary fiber content. And what you require nutri-

tionally may differ if you have other medical problems (like the American Heart Association recommends at least 1 g of omega-3 DHA/EPA for those with coronary heart disease). Rather, these steps are focused specifically on guidelines for healthy eating that will optimize brain function and restore critical elements of your brain chemistry that may become depleted as you deal with cancer, chemotherapy, and their aftermath.

STEP 5: DRINK DAILY FROM THE THREE BASIC BEVERAGE GROUPS—MILK, COFFEE, AND ALCOHOL (ESPECIALLY RED WINE) OR RED GRAPE JUICE

Milk

This beverage contains everything needed to keep us alive for months to years, even when no other food is consumed. Where else can you find such a natural supply of the following: (1) fluids, which are important for maintaining the right concentrations of electrolytes, such as sodium and potassium, for the electricity that flows in your brain and the right water pressure across cell membranes; (2) calcium, which is critical for the release of the neurotransmitters needed for communication from one neuron in your brain to the next; and (3) "whole" protein, which contains all the essential amino acids plus the fat-soluble vitamins A and D with which it's routinely fortified?

Coffee (or Other Caffeine Sources)

Caffeine provides the short-term benefits of increasing speed and accuracy of the cognitive processes, as well as enhancing a sense of well-being. Recent data also point to antioxidant, anti-inflammatory, and anti-amyloid activities of caffeine in the brain. (Coffee and tea, especially green tea, also contain other compounds besides caffeine that can contribute to health in a variety of ways.)

Alcohol

One to two drinks over the course of a day or a week can increase life expectancy as well as facilitate relaxation and the release of stress and tension, and diminish anxieties. Socially, a drink helps us loosen up just a bit; ultimately, that is good for your brain, too. All forms of ethanol are good in these respects, and red wine may be even better for you, probably because of the relatively high content of resveratrol and other antioxidants that come from the grape skins. Drinking to excess, however, may lead to the alcohol's killing more brain (and liver) cells than it is worth. If you have substance abuse or general addiction problems, or if you don't already drink, it may be better to stick to purple grape juice, which has a comparably high content of resveratrol and most other brain healthy compounds (pomegranate and cranberry juices are also good). See the boxed section below for a more detailed discussion of the potential risks and benefits of light to moderate alcohol consumption.

Alcohol and Cancer—Is There Really a Link?

You may have heard that there is an association between drinking alcohol and the incidence of some cancers, with the heaviest emphasis in the recent lay and professional literature directed toward different forms of breast cancers. How good is the evidence that daily consumption of one to two glasses of an alcoholic beverage actually can cause cancer, or cause a tumor to grow to the point detected by patients or their doctors?

First, no direct evidence exists that alcohol causes or exacerbates breast cancers in humans. The entire case is based upon statistical

analyses of epidemiologic data (which have pointed to at least a correlation between ongoing alcohol consumption and the incidence of
breast cancer), and "biologic plausibility" arguments derived from experiments conducted in vitro (test tubes and Petri dishes) or in
animals.

Nobody knows better than those in the breast cancer field how ultimately undependable those kinds of data and arguments are for es-
tablishing cause and effect. We witnessed this in 2002 when results
of one of the most significant randomized clinical trials (RCT) in U.S.
history (Women's Health Initiative, or WHI) disproved the assumption
based on seemingly overwhelming evidence that starting hormone
therapy (HT) in postmenopausal women did more good than harm
(see "What Went Wrong?" in Chapter 12).

But even if one were to accept the epidemiologic data at face
value and assume that the *entire* correlation was due to a causal link
flowing in only one direction (from alcohol to breast cancer), how
strong is that association anyway? The largest study to bear on that
question is the European Prospective Investigation into Cancer and
Nutrition (EPIC). It examined data collected on self-reported alcohol
consumption and cancer diagnoses in 274,688 middle-aged and elderly women from ten countries for up to 9.4 years (median 6.4
years).

During that time a total of 4,285 women were diagnosed with inva-
sive breast cancer. After the investigators adjusted statistical data to
account for body size, various sources of sex hormone exposure,
smoking status, and educational levels, they found that the incidence
of breast cancers among those women who drank no alcohol was

CONTINUES

1.39 percent. The incidence of breast cancers among those women who drank the alcohol equivalent of two glasses of wine per day (24 to 30 g ethanol) was 1.42 percent . . . that is, less than one-thirtieth of 1 percent increase. Those women who drank the equivalent of up to two to three glasses of wine per week (averaging up to 4.7 g ethanol/day) actually had a *lower* incidence of breast cancer than those women who drank no alcohol, though that difference was not statistically significant.[4]

If you wish to place *any* stock in such epidemiologic data, then take a look at the "big picture." As published in the highly esteemed journal *Annals of Internal Medicine*, researchers looked at the relative risk for death from coronary heart disease, cancer, and all causes—and how that risk correlated with beer, wine, and spirit consumption. Participants included about 25,000 Danish men and women, ages twenty to ninety-eight followed on average for ten years. And what the investigators found was that those who averaged up to one drink per day had a 2 percent increase in cancer deaths compared to those who drank no alcohol (not statistically significant). But they also demonstrated a highly significant 32 percent decrease in cardiovascular deaths, and an 18 percent decrease in the mortality rate overall. And for wine drinkers, specifically, the overall benefit of light alcohol consumption was even greater—associated with a 34 percent decrease in overall mortality![5]

Similarly, and even more pertinent to people with post-chemo brain, scientists published findings after following a group of women for thirty-four years—an extraordinarily long-term clinical follow-up of the same group of patients. At the end of that time, one out of nine suffered from dementia. The investigators found that those who drank wine had a 40 percent lower chance of becoming demented than those who did not. And those whose alcohol consumption consisted *only* of wine had a 70 percent *decreased* chance of developing dementia. But women who drank liquor had an increased chance of dementia of borderline statistical significance.[6] Given that we have encountered cancer centers where personnel actually counsel their patients to stop drinking "even a single glass of alcohol," one needs to ask whether that degree of alarm is actually justified by the scientific evidence.

Steps 6, 7, and 8: To Start at a Convenient Time Tomorrow

STEP 6: GET PHYSICAL

Being physically active is invaluable not only to your body in many general ways, but also specifically to your brain chemistry. Physical exercise reduces stress and stimulates your neuroendocrine system in a healthy way (see Chapter 16). So:

Exercise your heart and lungs (with pulse-elevating aerobic exercise) three or four times each week.

Exercise at least some of your major skeletal muscles (arms, legs, chest, back, and abdomen) at least two times a week.

Do fun things that involve physical activity—as often as you can fit them in and certainly on days that you don't otherwise get your cardio or exercise your muscles. For example, you might want to do one of these things: walking, biking, hiking, swimming, tennis, gardening, or washing the car. Just get moving and enjoy yourself!

And, speaking of that, there is no physical outlet more effective in helping people to enjoy themselves, from a neurologic point of view, than engaging in sexual activity.

It shouldn't be hard to do fun things that involve physical activity. But if it is for you, then consider talking to your doctor. Ask to be evaluated for anergia (no energy), anhedonia (no interest in pleasurable activities), and/or depression (which can cause both of the above). Therapies might include bupropion to boost your dopaminergic reward pathways if you have either or both of the latter two problems, and supplementary therapy with a catecholaminergic stimulant (e.g., methylphenidate, dexmethylphenidate, or modafinil) could help with any or all three. Refer to Chapter 15 regarding these neurostimulant drugs.

About Sex

Human beings have survived during hundreds of thousands of years of evolution through natural selection (often described as "survival of the fittest") and sexual selection (mating opportunities for the "hottest"). We are biologically driven to get as many of our genes as possible into the next generation. From an evolutionary point of view, this is our *raison d'être*. And one of the ways your brain makes sure you know it is by devoting a significant portion of your hypothalamus to regulating the magnitude and orientation of your sex drive. You are also wired to receive very powerful input from your sex organs into the reward pathways (what used to be called the "pleasure center") of your brain. Sexual stimulation is a much more potent stimulus of our neurological reward pathways than even a runner's high.

STEP 7: GET A MENTAL AND/OR SOCIAL WORKOUT

Stay engaged mentally, socially—and intellectually. Not only does keeping yourself stimulated deflect your attention away from ruminating, or obsessive thoughts, but also it all adds to deepening your interests and the dimensions of who you are and how you relate socially. One way is to keep up with current events. Use news sources where *you* are in control of the information stream, such as by surfing the Internet or perusing broad-topic weekly magazines such as *Newsweek* or *Time*. Avoid TV and tabloid sources that spoon-feed sensational and distressing (depressing!) information.

STEP 8: APPRECIATE THE BIG PICTURE WITH
A GOOD MOOD AND ATTITUDE

Just as the condition of your body strongly influences the status of your brain chemistry (and, consequently, your mind), the status of your mind strongly influences the condition of your body, including your brain chemistry. Your brain chemistry exercises control of your body through the neuroendocrine system, the autonomic nervous system (sympathetic and parasympathetic; see Chapter 16), and through voluntary peripheral nervous systems. Brain chemistry also influences how well you think and what kind of mood you're in. The bottom line is this: What you do to and with your mind is inestimably important to what happens to your body (including your brain), which in turn feeds back upon your cognitive status.

Writers and scholars have long recognized the intimate relationship between attitudes and outcomes. The poet John Milton observed in the seventeenth century, "The mind is its own place, and in itself can make a heaven of hell, and a hell of heaven." William James, a nineteenth-century pioneer of the modern field of psychology said,

"The greatest discovery of my generation is that a human being can alter his life by altering his attitude." And even long before the practice of cognitive therapy was invented, Dale Carnegie, the author of the self-help classic *How to Win Friends and Influence People*, observed in the early twentieth century, "It isn't what you have, or who you are, or where you are, or what you are doing that makes you happy or unhappy. It is what you think about." Decades later, the founders of cognitive theory echoed that concept, which today is the basis of empirically well-validated cognitive therapy techniques.

Feeling grateful is also important to cognitive well-being. In a series of clever experiments at a large, public university, subjects logged sincere thoughts of gratitude into a journal on a daily and/or weekly basis. The researchers found that taking time to focus your thoughts on people and things for which you are grateful could diminish physical symptoms, as well as significantly increase mood, optimism, and the number of hours spent exercising each week.[7]

Finally, a number of studies support that laughter is good medicine, so cultivate both a sense of perspective and a sense of humor by trying to see the lighter sides of even serious situations, and by seeking out sources of entertainment and people who are funny. Some cancer support organizations even hold laughter sessions.

A Word of General Advice

STEP 9: AVOID DOCTORS, DRUGS, AND HOSPITALS

Perhaps you've heard the expression: "When all you have is a hammer, everything looks like a nail." All the more so for specialists (a general practitioner is someone who *thinks* he knows what you have, and a specialist is someone who thinks you *have* what he knows), so the more time you spend around doctors, the more likely you are to get "nailed" . . . for example, with tests that are ordered, to follow up on other tests that weren't really necessary in the first place . . . or medicines prescribed that take the place of what you could and should be accomplishing with lifestyle changes.

If you urgently need medical care or if you are in treatment for cancer, the advice does not apply to you.[8] But otherwise, ask yourself this: Do I really need to see a doctor about this? Often people go to doctors when they really don't need to be there. They go because they are feeling run down or because they have a low-grade temperature: Unless you're undergoing chemotherapy or radiation therapy and you are immunosupressed, there is typically no urgency. Give your immune system a few days to do its job. Others see doctors for reassurance. But you don't need calming words from physicians. (They generally don't have enough time to really talk to you, anyway, as you likely found if you've ever tried to have a conversation with one!) You will be far better off talking to an understanding friend or family member or to those in a support group who have shared the same experiences.

And hospitals are no place to be when you are already ill; they are depressing places, and depression can impair recovery. It is no great secret that people can get even sicker in hospitals, sometimes even hastening their death when seriously ill. Infections can spread from patients to hospital employees and back to patients. The facility itself is contaminated with antibiotic-resistant bacteria. There are just a whole slew of reasons to stay away. If you must be there, get in, and get out.

Of course, it's always better to avoid getting a serious medical problem than to have to get treatment for one, so as Alpert suggests in his eighth prescription for "health, happiness, and longevity," preventive health care is an exception to the above. *Do* get your prostate gland or your breasts and cervix examined as regularly as recommended, bite the bullet and submit to a colonoscopy if you are at least fifty or if it has been a decade since your last one. And consider getting vaccinated against the flu, etc., if you fall within a significantly at-risk group.

CHAPTER 20

Summary of the Nine Steps and Worksheet

Following the suggestions listed in Chapter 19 will help you reenergize your brain. After cancer and chemotherapy, it may feel as if you're trying to run your 25-watt brain with only enough battery power to generate 10 to 15 watts. And just as other batteries tend to rust and corrode when you don't use or recharge them, your brain's electrical circuits—that are normally wide open, allowing your thoughts to fly through—may have become laden during chemotherapy with a kind of functional rust, slowing your thought-processing to a crawl.

The nine-step program will help you regain your pre-chemo level of cerebral functioning by:

• enabling your body to supply more power to your brain cells, which in turn will infuse your neuronal circuitry with more of the energy needed to process your thoughts,

- increasing your capacity to use this newly infused energy to greater advantage by boosting your brain's ability—especially for carrying information along the neuronal circuits pertinent to restoring high-level cognitive function, and
- retaining in those circuits what you are learning, as you go forward.

To accomplish these goals:

Steps 1 and 2 (*a productive focus and a regulated clock*) will optimize the general functioning of your brain, so that it works efficiently during both waking and sleeping hours.

Steps 3, 4, and 5 (*eat foods and drink beverages that do good things for your brain*) are all about charging up your batteries by directly supplying your brain's immediate chemical environment with plentiful sources of vitamins and minerals, proteins and omega-3s, antioxidants, and neurostimulants. They ensure that the right kinds of chemical energy flow vigorously through healthy vessels.

Steps 6, 7, and 8 (*give your body, mind, and spirit all they need to thrive*) are for reaping the fruits of the positive brain chemistry changes.

Step 9 (*use doctors, drugs, and hospitals for [only] the right things*) is, finally, about keeping it all healthy since your brain is influenced by the condition of the rest of your body. So take advantage of proven preventive health measures. Get the medical care you really need while avoiding what you don't.

Getting Started—The First Two Weeks

Now that you know *what* to do each day, the *only* thing left is to actually do it! Take advantage of the point-by-point checklist in Table 20.1. We suggest you make fifteen photocopies. You can use one copy

TABLE 20.1: Daily Checklist: A Nine-Step Program

☐ 1) focus on (only) the things I can do something about

☐ 2) keep my brain's biological clock running on time

☐ 3) get 4-5 servings of fruits and vegetables . . . or at least a multivitamin pill, and . . .

☐ 4) no less than 60g protein + 0.4 g (400 mg) DHA/EPA omega-3; no more than 60 g fat (20 g saturated)

☐ 5) drink milk, coffee, and alcohol* (or suitable equivalents)

☐ 6) give my muscles a workout and/or have physical fun every day (and if I can't or won't, see a doc to give my neurotransmitters a more direct lift)

☐ 7) feed my head with information that is interesting to me, and share it with others

☐ 8) anticipate the best possible outcomes from my main action(s) of this day (but be set for the worst by having a "Plan B" ready . . . and by cultivating a "big picture" perspective)

☐ 9) get preventive health care when I'm due . . . but cancel/don't make doctor appointments I can avoid!**

* (grape juice for alcoholics and teetotalers)
** (that is, see my doctor when I need to . . . but not when I don't)

tonight for the top two items, and the rest will keep you on track for the next two weeks. Check off the first eight items daily as you accomplish them. Step number nine is there to serve you as needed.

To remind yourself about the details regarding any of these items, refer back to the corresponding numbered subsections in the preceding chapter.

Making It All Work

After two weeks, page through your daily lists and look for patterns. Take a moment to reflect. Where did you fall short? Where did you succeed, and what did you do to make that happen? (Do not skip this last part, as looking at what you did *right* means not being hyperfocused on what you did wrong, which in itself would be bad for brain chemistry.)

If you accomplished the top eight steps routinely, then keep up the good work! But you may not have hit your mark every time. If not, determine why and, if needed, tailor the program to your individual situation and beliefs. If after four good-faith tries (i.e., eight weeks of following the above) you still are not getting the results from the program that you believe you should, see the authors' notes.

CHAPTER 21

Future Directions

So what does the next decade promise? That we will treat smarter, with more specific treatments and vaccines that target cancer cells while leaving healthy cells intact. We will decipher even further how our brains react to diseases and therapies. And we will better understand the mechanisms behind cognitive dysfunction.

Like a maddening puzzle with multiple chambers, there are questions within questions. Here is what we know. It appears that a substantial portion of people—maybe one-third—who are diagnosed with cancer show cognitive impairment on neuropsychological tests, even *before* treatment of any kind. Many of these same patients show even *greater* cognitive impairment after chemotherapy, and additional patients show measurable cognitive impairment only *after* chemotherapy. How do you explain that? How do you sort out which aspects of cognitive impairment are due to cancer, which are due to chemotherapy, and which are an interaction of the two?

It is not easy. In an ideal experimental design, we would follow thousands of people over a period of years to show how their mental abilities change over time. We would start not at the time of diagnosis, but before a single cancer cell had taken hold. We would test memory and concentration skills to establish a baseline. At diagnosis, we would retest to see if their functioning had changed. After chemotherapy we would do the same, and several times more through recovery, and for years following.

> *"The first time I had chemo and felt the red liquid running up my vein, I asked the nurse about my brain, my brain cells, and all that, and she answered that it didn't go into your brain. I remember thinking that was kind of nuts. How could anyone tell me that those toxins don't go to your brain, that they turn around and don't go there! The best thing that can come out of all of us telling our stories is that doctors can say, 'Yes, it's true, you are destroying brain cells.'"*
>
> —Jackson Hunsicker, breast cancer, diagnosed in 2000 at age fifty-one. (Treatment: lumpectomy, radiation. Chemo: cyclophosphamide, doxorubicin and paclitaxel.)

Of course, we won't know in advance who will win the raffle and remain cognitively unscathed, and who will not. But just by addressing the questions, some of the riddle unfolds. We know that many cancer survivors experience cognitive problems that are debilitating. We also know that chemotherapy does not cross the blood-brain barrier in very high concentrations . . . at least when the blood-brain barrier is healthy. So then if chemotherapy is not directly causing the cognitive decline, what is?

Could It Be the Cytokines?

A leading hypothesis in the field is that a family of molecules called *cytokines* may be responsible. Cytokines are inflammatory molecules that are generally produced by white blood cells or sometimes cancer cells. Our bodies pump out these cytokines in response to injury or infection, and some can freely cross the blood-brain barrier. It may be that chemotherapy agents and/or steroids and other medications bundled with treatment or the cancer cells themselves, are causing this cytokine release that can be toxic to our brain tissue.

A BODY OF MESSAGES

There are many different types of cytokines, and they serve specific functions. Some are called interleukins, and others are called interferons. They fight infections and stimulate other cells of the immune system into action. Think of cytokines as messages that are sent from one cell to another or from one cell to lots of other cells. They are also what make you feel sick when you have the flu, as the interleukins and other cytokines flood your bloodstream as a consequence. You might feel nauseous, for example, because cytokines are telling you to lose your appetite. Your fever may be enhancing the ability of your immune system to fight off a virus. Your lethargy directs you to sit or lie quietly while your body conserves energy to be used in fighting off the bug.

So your viral infection is not necessarily what is causing your symptoms directly. The symptoms reflect how your body is reacting in response to cytokine signals. That is why so many different illnesses have symptoms of fever, nausea, and fatigue in common. They are included in what scientists often refer to as "sick syndrome." Some of the symptoms of depression can be part of that as well.

DELIVERING MISCHIEF

But as important as cytokines are, once they cross the blood-brain barrier, they can damage brain tissue or affect nerve function. In fact, in published studies reviewed in the *Lancet* in 2004, the authors reported that some cancer patients treated with the cytokine interferon-alpha demonstrated impaired memory and concentration and speech problems.[1] Others treated with the cytokine interleukin 2 showed deficits in spatial working memory and planning. They also found that fatigue was reported in 70 to 100 percent of patients who received interferon, depending on schedule and dose. Cancer survivors who are one or two years out from diagnosis may have cytokine levels that are elevated by factors of ten or even by a hundred! [2]

Overall, if you have high cytokine levels you are more likely to experience fatigue and cognitive dysfunction than people without elevated cytokines. We also know that cytokines used as drugs can cause side effects such as low mood, sleep disturbance, apathy, and impaired thinking.

Cytokines may very well be the most critical component in that cascade of events that leads to "chemo brain." If we find that post-chemotherapy impairment is conclusively associated with these molecules, then we can aim to develop drugs that disarm or tie up cytokines before they slip into the brain, or that protect brain tissue from their damaging effects.

The Role of Brain Imaging

We can now do direct imaging of the living human brain in ways that allow us to directly visualize illnesses of the mind. MR and CT scans give us high-resolution images of brain structure, allowing us, from outside the head, to detect things in the brain that are less than a sixteenth of an inch in diameter. MR imaging can also be used in a functional mode, to look at changes occurring in brain activity over a period of a few seconds.

Neuronuclear imaging tools, positron emission tomography (PET), and single-photon emission computed tomography (SPECT) are especially versatile for examining the function and chemistry of the brain. They enable us to measure how quickly blood passes through each region of the brain, the rate at which each region of our brain uses the sugar glucose (its main source of fuel), the consumption of oxygen, the uptake of amino acids from which neurotransmitters and proteins are synthesized, and how well molecules have penetrated the blood-brain barrier. These images can, in turn, help us diagnose and treat conditions as varied as brain tumors, epilepsy, and neurodegenerative disorders such as Alzheimer's and Parkinson's disease, as well as examine changes in the brain associated with mood disorders and cognitive decline. Even more pertinent, these tools help us measure diminished brain function associated with alterations in cognition and mood after chemotherapy, region by region through the brain. With them we can monitor improvements in brain function that occur with treatments and/or with the healing power of time.

CAPTURING YOUR *NORMAL*

So far, we have seen associations between cognition, cancer therapies, and brain metabolism in small groups of patients. If we are able to confirm the same kinds of associations in larger studies (now underway), those findings could lead to bolder approaches in patient care. One strategy, as described earlier, would offer patients a more complete PET scan prior to chemotherapy. Currently doctors order a "whole-body" PET/CT that scans from the mid-thigh to the base of the skull to stage certain cancers or check for new tumors. Using both PET and CT on the same device allows doctors to see function (PET) and structure (CT). Patients with many types of tumors commonly undergo these scans, including those with lymphoma, melanoma, lung, colorectal, esophageal, liver, pancreatic, brain, ovarian, and breast cancers. By spending a few extra minutes in the scanner, patients could have the device go all the way to the top of their heads (instead of stopping at the skull base). It could take pictures of the brain and measure its metabolism, region by region. That baseline of how the brain functions prior to treatment would serve as a point for comparison with each subsequent scan.

SCANS AND RADIATION

Some people worry about additional radiation, especially to the brain. But with whole-body PET, it does not work like that. Yes, the CT part of the scanner does deliver some extra radiation, but it can be a low dose. In fact, the next generation of PET scanners for the brain—a combination of PET/MRI—will use no radiation to take the structural pictures. The small amount of radiolabeled tracer compound you receive for a PET scan already circulates everywhere in the body, including the brain. So why not take pictures of that while the tracer is already in your body and your body is already in the scanner?

INTERVENING *BEFORE* YOU FORGET

The beauty of PET information, especially for people on long-term therapy, is that with progressive neurologic conditions, the scans are so sensitive that weeks or months or years before you even develop symptoms, you can see changes in brain metabolism. With that information, you can potentially intervene *before* you start to experience problems with concentration or memory or word retrieval. In the future, doctors will explain to patients that scans are also a tool to *prevent* permanent cognitive damage. Once problems show up in neuropsychological tests, that window has passed. You would then be focusing on strategies to compensate for your deficits.

What doctors and their patients want, of course, is the best possible outcome from treatment with the fewest side effects, especially those that might significantly impact your life. Perhaps you are someone whose basal ganglia metabolism (an area of the brain important for translating thought into action) prior to treatment is already lower than average. Your doctor might consider you at increased risk for suffering cognitive impairment should you receive chemotherapy combined with antihormonal therapy. But what if you have lots of basal ganglia metabolism to spare? The added risk of cognitive impairment with combination therapy might be less of an issue.

Using scans to monitor potential risks is not a new idea. Oncologists, for instance, routinely order a different type (called MUGA, multiple gated acquisition scans) to measure heart function in patients who are on doxorubicin-type compounds and/or the targeted therapy trastuzumab (Herceptin).

Designer Chemotherapy

In the future, medical imaging will be an important key to personalized treatment, not only for cancers, but also across many disease groups. Right now it does not work that way. How and why a patient receives one drug versus another is largely dependent on the results of randomized drug therapy trials. Hundreds of people may be given drug regimen A during these trials, while hundreds more may be given drug regimen B. Let's say 55 percent of the people assigned to regimen A respond, but 70 percent respond to B. It will be B that becomes the drug regimen of choice. Yet what about that significant group—30 percent—who did not respond to B? They may have been better off with regimen A.

CHEMOSENSITIVITY TESTING

In Vitro (In Test Tubes)

Recognizing this, in previous decades scientists had attempted to individualize treatments for patients based on in vitro screening for effectiveness. No one wants to suffer through harsh side effects, including nerve damage and cognitive dysfunction, especially if the toxins are not going to kill or control the cancer in the first place. So scientists worked on developing *chemotherapy sensitivity and resistance assays.* After surgery or biopsy, cells from patients' tumors are sent to a lab and divided into multiple small samples, which researchers expose to various chemotherapy agents. These assays are designed to test whether the cancer cells will respond to the drug or resist it and continue to grow.

Doctors have long used this approach to fight infectious diseases. A urine sample from someone with a bladder infection, for example, may end up divided in several plastic wells. Each may contain a different type or dose of antibiotic. Hopefully, the experiment comes up with the best drug regimen for that individual patient. But unfortunately, for the purpose of picking chemotherapy regimens for tumors, these assays are not dependable. They do have strong, negative predictive value. That is, if they do not work in the plastic well, they usually will not work in the person. But they have only weak positive predictive value, meaning regimens that work great in at-

tacking the tumor cells in the lab can end up being completely inef-
fective in controlling the cancer in the patients' bodies.

In Vivo (In the Body)

Obviously, the best way to see if the drugs are working is to determine
if they are killing the cancer inside your body. We will want to know
if the chemo is actually getting to the right cells. Is the concentration
high enough in the tumor cells to kill the cancer, but low enough in
the normal tissues to leave healthy organs intact? Does the drug stay
with the tumor long enough to be effective?

Often oncologists can't tell until the chemicals have had a chance
to do their job (or not). So you sit in the doctor's office, enduring a
close, personal relationship with an IV line to your vein. After several
weeks or months of these visits, you may be sent for a PET/CT scan
and worry yourself sick until you get the results. By then your hair
has fallen out. Vomiting has become a way of life. You can no longer
feel the bottom of your feet. And, yes, you are tired of finding the
ketchup bottle in the freezer.

What if it were possible to see which drugs would be most effective
by testing them in the body prior to treatment, kind of like a color-
safe fabric test for the wash? What if the amounts were so small—
just one-hundredth or one-thousandth of what you would normally
get—that they would not cause side effects? What if you could find
out the results within days?

That is where we are headed now. In our lab at UCLA, for example,
we conducted studies using PET scans for predicting the effectiveness
of each of the major classes of cytotoxic chemotherapy agents used
to fight breast, as well as many other, cancers. We tagged each of
these drugs with a radioactive isotope of fluorine so that we could

trace their distributions in mice implanted with human breast cancers, using a small-animal version of a PET scanner. After just a tiny dose, much smaller than would cause any known side effects, we were able to measure how much of it got into the tumors, how quickly it got there, and how long it stayed. We were able to predict whether the tumors would grow or decrease after getting a big dose of each chemotherapy compound.

If and when such research is fully translated into human use, patients could get PET scans with these kinds of tracer drugs. Potentially, we would know which chemotherapy agent or combination of agents work for an individual and which do not *before* the large side-effect-producing doses are taken.

In addition, we could take pictures of the brain to say which of these drug regimens are most risky to the cognitive function of an individual patient.

Bringing Drugs to Market

Until then, we will rely on the creativity of scientists and other experts to develop pharmaceutical and non-drug approaches. Their work will help us neutralize the bad effects. Already there are small trials of drugs like modafinil and other stimulants. But even these promising drugs must still be tested in larger-scale trials before the FDA can approve them for the specific treatment of post-chemo brain. We may see other compounds, currently used for dementia, modified to benefit people with chemo-related dysfunction. Alternative therapies from herbs and roots as well have entered the mainstream as the literature grows about their effectiveness. After all, many of our pharmaceuticals actually began in the natural world. Out of the 120 or so prescription drugs used to treat cancer, about 90 were derived from plants.[3] Paclitaxel, now commonly used in the treatment of breast cancer, is one example. It is isolated from the bark of the Pacific yew tree.

Are My Memories Gone Forever?

Not necessarily. We see some surprising recoveries in patients referred for brain imaging whose cognitive changes look like they could be a precursor to Alzheimer's disease. When carefully selected, many—about 80 percent—will, in fact, eventually develop dementia. The other 20 percent will either remain stable, or their changes will reverse. We don't know for sure what triggers recovery in many patients. But something clicks in the biochemistry of their brains. In some cases, it may have something to do with those cytokines, an anti-inflammatory response, mediated by compounds in the diet, medications, stress reduction, and/or their own immune systems.

If you asked a team of scientists from the Massachusetts Institute of Technology whether more severe learning and memory deficits could be reversed, they would also respond affirmatively. They were able to restore memories in mice that had been genetically altered to develop cognitive decline and brain damage similar to what is seen in Alzheimer's disease. The implications were stunning.

An initial step came when Li-Huei Tsai, Ph.D., a professor of neuroscience at MIT, and her colleagues engineered these mice to produce p25—a protein implicated in Parkinson's and Alzheimer's disease. The protein causes brain atrophy, but the gene coding for it can be switched on or off by feeding the mice certain antibiotics. Two key experiments came next. Both were reported in 2007 in the journal *Nature*.[4] In one, the scientists took these mice—before switching on the gene—and conditioned them to associate a specific structure with a mild electric shock. The idea was that they would learn to freeze in place when they saw it. The researchers also set

235

up a water maze, putting the mice in a tiny swimming pool. Mice don't like water. So they quickly learned to get to a platform submerged out of sight.

Tsai and her team gave the mice four weeks to encode what they had learned into long-term memory and then "switched on" the gene for p25. The mice experienced severe neuron loss in their forebrains and forgot what they had learned. A few weeks later, the scientists started the enrichment part of the study. While some mice continued to live in normal cages, others were housed in a special cage with an exercise treadmill, climbing devices, tunnels, and a variety of colorful toys. All were changed daily.

Then the scientists retested the cognitively impaired group. Remarkably, the mice housed in the enriched environment recovered what they had learned. The other mice whose p25 had been "switched on" but were not given enrichment did not.

Later, researchers examined the brains of the enriched mice. It was not that new neurons had formed to replace what had been destroyed. Rather, remaining neurons had compensated for the loss.

As Li-Huei Tsai commented, "This recovery of long-term memory was really the most remarkable finding. It suggests that memories are not really erased in such disorders as Alzheimer's, but that they are rendered inaccessible and can be recovered."[5]

Her message is profoundly hopeful for all people with cognitive impairment due to a wide range of causes, from Alzheimer's disease to post-chemo brain. The point is that someone's cognitive abilities could be decimated by pathological changes that are irreversible, like neuronal cell death. But the right interventions, from drugs to environmental enrichment, could restore even memories that had seemed irretrievably lost.

As with other health-related conditions, prevention beats intervention. The ultimate objective shared by all of us is stopping cancer from occurring in the first place through adequate screening, development of anti-cancer vaccinations, and healthful lifestyle choices. And what is "plan B" for those cases we cannot prevent? To treat patients with therapies that make them well without harming the health and functioning of their brains and other normal tissues.

Meanwhile, the information, recommendations, and resources described in this book will help you restore your mental agility so that you are as capable after chemo as you were before it. You *can* improve your mind and spirit. You *can* regain your focus. And as you use this book, you'll be armed with the best tools available for tapping into the power of your brain to bring out the old you who's been waiting inside.

Authors' Notes

DAN SILVERMAN You may be wondering why a book about the effects of chemotherapy on the brain has so much material about two cancers in particular, namely breast and lymphoma. This is not, as far as we know, because these two cancers have any special relationship to the brain, but simply because they are cancers where people often receive chemotherapy at an early enough stage of disease that they become long-term survivors, even completely cured. (For many other cancers, in contrast, chemotherapy is often reserved for more advanced stages of disease.) As a consequence, relatively large numbers of people who had chemotherapy for lymphoma or breast cancer years ago have participated in these cognitive studies, providing us with the most compelling evidence for the chemotherapy/brain connection.

As a physician who frequently sees patients undergoing (or who have previously undergone) chemotherapy for all kinds of cancer, and as a scientist who continues to research methods to prevent and treat adverse effects of chemotherapy, I encourage you to let me know not only what you found helpful in this book, but also what has given (and perhaps continues to give) you the most difficulty. Feel free to send any questions or comments you may have directly to my office e-mail address below. We will respond to you individually (eventually!), even if the reply is, as it may often be, "At this point, we just don't have a clear answer for that." Your messages will remain confidential. No identifying information from their contents will ever be made public without your explicit approval.

IDELLE DAVIDSON As a journalist and someone who believes we all have the right to engage fully in our medical care, I hope you will continue to send me your stories as well as strategies or tips that helped you lift the fog after chemo. Only with your permission will I share them.

To protect the confidentiality of those whose stories appear in *Your Brain After Chemo*, we have changed a few names and sometimes other identifying information.

Thank you.

—*Dan Silverman, M.D., Ph.D.*
(e-mail: dansilverman@rocketmail.com)
—*Idelle Davidson*
(e-mail: IdelleDavidson@gmail.com)

Acknowledgments

DAN SILVERMAN Thanks are due to a number of people who have contributed to the creation of this book, directly or indirectly—including co-workers and other colleagues who work in medical, scientific and literary circles; patients whom I've seen clinically and others whom I have not but who have nevertheless generously shared their personal stories; family members and friends; and people whose contributions have come from two or more of these roles or escape simple categorization altogether—only a few of whom will be mentioned here.

Among those most directly involved with this project, I would like to express my gratitude, first of all, to my co-author Idelle Davidson, for the many invaluable roles she assumed in bringing to fruition a work of this kind, beginning with its original conception. Over the two years of our collaboration on it, she has been everything from creative author of her own material and critical editor of mine, to multitalented (and multitasking) interviewer, investigator, business-woman, and intellectual property consultant. . . . Plus, as nearly all of the published works for which I've previously served as author or co-author have been directed toward readers who are professionally immersed in evaluating, treating, and/or scientifically investigating clinically pertinent aspects of the mind and body, this present effort has benefited immensely from Idelle's skills and experience in bringing medically oriented writings to readers who are themselves experiencing the profound effects of the medical conditions upon which the writings are focused.

We are in turn indebted to our agent Carol Mann, and our editors Matthew Lore and Wendy Francis, who have been indispensable guides and colleagues during the process of moving this effort forward—from being something abstractly in our heads to something concretely in your hand. I personally wish to thank them for their understanding of the problems posed by my need to divide attentions among the oft-competing demands of contributing to a writing project of this magnitude while concomitantly fulfilling my ongoing clinical, scientific, and educational responsibilities.

I also wish to acknowledge the creative artistry of my research associate (and Aerial Showgirl extraordinaire) Cheri Geist and of my younger daughter Ariel Silverman, for devoting their ideas and talents to producing illustrations for this book, as well as the conscientiously applied transcriptional skills contributed to this project by my daughter Kalina Silverman.

I would further like to thank my friend and colleague Guesh Cuan for valuable discussions in which she offered her unique perspective into treating the types of problems often suffered by patients post-chemo, based upon an intimate knowledge of traditional Chinese medical practices and effects of cancer/therapy on the brain, in combination with her experiences as a researcher and student also of Western medicine as it is practiced in both the United States and China.

There are other people, perhaps less directly involved in this project, though not less directly involved in my professional or personal life during the time I was working on it, to whom I am deeply indebted: my chemo-expert colleagues at the David Geffen School of Medicine, neuropsychologist Steve Castellon, and oncologist Patti Ganz, who continually serve to educate me on important areas related to post-chemo brain well beyond my own scope of knowledge; my friends and research associates who have worked with me in the Neuronuclear Imaging Section of the Ahmanson Biological Imaging Division at UCLA Medical Center on chemotherapy- and hormone-related brain effects, providing the basis for much of my firsthand knowledge of the corresponding scientific aspects of this book— Betty Pio, Cheri Geist, Jasmine Lai, Christine Dy, Natalie Htet, Vicky Lau, and Erin Siu; and my wife, Wei Chen, for her patience and support throughout this period that I've been pouring what otherwise could have been much valuable "family time" into completion of this work.

IDELLE DAVIDSON Writing this book has been the most stimulating kind of brain exercise. For two years I have held a ticket to a front-row seat at seminars where my co-author is the featured speaker and I am the only attendee. It is because of my collaboration with Dan Silverman that I learned about the evolution of the human brain and what sets us apart from other primates. It is from our countless conversations that I developed an appreciation for the humanness of emotion, nurturing, personality, and abstract reasoning. When Dan talks about the complexity of this gelatin-like organ we call the brain, you can almost see his own neurons firing. His speech quickens; his ideas race. He has a passion for understanding how and why we think, and I thank him for sharing it with me.

I extend my appreciation as well to our agent, the capable Carol Mann, who in the time it takes to sneeze found a home for our manuscript at Da Capo Press. There, it was our delight to work with editors Matthew Lore and Wendy Francis.

A multitude of other medical specialists served as resources. I am grateful to the following: Dr. Tim Ahles and Dr. Denise Correa at Memorial Sloan-Kettering Cancer Center; Dr. Debra Barton at the Mayo Clinic; Dr. Catherine Bender at the University of Pittsburgh; Dr. Pauline Maki at the University of Illinois at Chicago; Dr. Natalie Rasgon at Stanford University; Dr. Robert Ferguson at the Eastern Maine Medical Center; Dr. Ian Tannock at the University of Toronto; Dr. Sadhna Kohli at the University of Rochester; Dr. Bernadine Cimprich at the University of Michigan; Dr. Jeffrey Scott Wefel, Dr. Christina Meyes, and Dr. Lorenzo Cohen at the University of Texas MD Anderson Cancer Center; Dr. Arti Hurria at City of Hope; Dr. Ann Partridge at Dana-Farber Cancer Institute; Dr. Cathy Levenson at Florida State University; Dr. Sara Lazar at Massachusetts General Hospital; and Dr. Artemis Simopoulos, author of *The Omega Diet*. Additional thanks to the UCLA contingent: Dr. Linda Ercoli, Dr. Steven Castellon, Dr. Stanley Korenman, Dr. Julienne Bower, Dr. Kenneth A. Conklin, and Sherry Goldman, R.N., C.N.P., director of patient services at the Revlon/UCLA Breast Center.

Sherry Goldman deserves singling out. Not only did she contribute to the book, but she performed a particular kindness for me when I was in treatment and most vulnerable. She may not remember the circumstances, but I will never forget. Thank you also to Sara Goldberger of Gilda's Club, and Janet Colantuono of Hurricane Voices. Janet graciously allowed us to reprint results from her survey "Cognitive Changes Related to Cancer Treatment." I am also grateful to Malcolm Schultz and Michael States of the Wellness Community in West Los Angeles, and Nancy Raymon and Donna Farris of Healing Odyssey. I am a proud graduate of their programs.

It was my great honor to talk with dozens of cancer survivors across the United States and internationally—men and women and their families who entrusted me with their poignant, sometimes sad, but always hopeful stories. To Patrick and Cam and Susan and Michael and Erica and Dawn and Carol and Richard and Jackson and J and Zizi and so many others whose voices comprise this book, I thank you for sharing your experiences, for your candor, for your caring that others know they are not alone.

To the award-winning artist Dave Coverly of Speed Bump, thank you for allowing us use of your cartoon, "Tip of the Tongue."

I am grateful to several friends: Dr. Joyce Parker who offered counsel (and humor) when I needed it most as we walked along the bluffs overlooking the Pacific Ocean; fellow writers Pam Leven and Patty Salier for their wit and observations; and Dr. Rhona Schreck for her always–accessible scientific mind.

I would especially like to thank novelist Kathryn (Kate) A. Graham who took time from her own writing career to transcribe most of the interviews, all with perfection.

Many authors thank their families for their love and support. I understand why. In my husband Peter's case, he served as emotional stabilizer and reasoned voice when the weight of research, reporting, and writing seemed more than I could lift. Thank you, Peter. I won't share all my private thoughts on these public pages, but you know. Our two sons Ben and Matt deserve credit as well for contributing in other important ways. Ben, an MBA finance whiz, computed hundreds of entries of U.S. Department of Agriculture raw data about omega-3 and omega-6 fatty acids into usable reports so that I could integrate the material in the manuscript. That raw data, by the way, was very kindly generated specifically for us by nutritionist Linda Lemar of the USDA Nutrient Data Laboratory.

Matt, a Ph.D. student at Stanford School of Medicine, provided me with the majority of the scientific journal articles that you see referenced in the text. Not only did he somehow find the time between his graduate studies and research work (and running his own chewing gum company) to pull these articles for me, but he was just late-night calls away when I needed the similes that lead to clarity: " . . . so, dendritic cells are like the generals that train the troops."

I would also like to thank my mother, Taube, my mother-in-law, Florence, and my sister and brother (and best friends forever) Carole and Charles for checking in with me almost daily during the writing process and for being there always. To the rest of my family, thank you. I value and appreciate you all.

Appendix
Resources

Cognitive Training Programs
Memory and Attention Adaptation Training: MAAT

Robert J. Ferguson, Ph.D., Eastern Maine Medical Center,
Maine Rehabilitation Outpatient Center, 905 Union St.,
Bangor, ME 04401

Phone (207) 973-4037

Fax (207) 973-8276

An individualized cognitive training program for cancer survivors
that was designed by Robert J. Ferguson, Ph.D., an adjunct assistant professor of psychiatry at Dartmouth Medical School and a
clinical health psychologist at Eastern Maine Medical Center in
Bangor, Maine. The program has been developed with funding by
the Office of Cancer Survivorship, National Cancer Institute,
and the Lance Armstrong Foundation.

Software and Online Training

PositScience Brain Fitness Program

www.positscience.com

Phone (415) 394-3100

Toll free (800) 514-3961

....

Mindfit Back on Track

www.cognifit.com

Toll free: (866) 669-6223

....

HappyNeuron.com

www.happy-neuron.com

Toll free (800) 560-0966 x 1

....

Brain Games (a handheld, electronic game)

www.radicagames.com/brain-games.php

(800) 803-9611

Emotional and Psychological Support

Many major medical centers offer programs for cancer survivors, including lectures by cancer experts, nutrition classes and workshops on stress reduction. Check with the medical center closest to you.

....

Healing Odyssey

www.healingodyssey.org

Phone: (949) 951-3930

Provides three-day weekend retreats for women cancer survivors in the mountains of Malibu, California. An oncology nurse specialist and an oncology social worker along with a staff of specially trained camp counselors run the program in a psychologically supportive environment. Many graduates of these retreats credit Healing Odyssey for helping them through a difficult time in their lives. Based on ability to pay.

Young Survival Coalition YSC

www.youngsurvival.org

Phone (646) 257-3000

Toll free (877) YSC-1011

Through "action, advocacy, and awareness," YSC supports the unique concerns of women forty and under affected by breast cancer.

The Wellness Community

www.thewellnesscommunity.org

Phone: (202) 659-9709

Toll-free: (888) 793-WELL

Founded in 1982, The Wellness Community is an international non-profit organization that provides free support, education, and hope to people with cancer and their loved ones, in one hundred locations worldwide and online. Lots of classes, including meditation, yoga, etc.

Gilda's Club

www.gildasclub.org

Phone: (888) GILDA-4-U

A worldwide organization that offers "cancer support for the whole family, the whole time." Gilda's Club was named for *Saturday Night Live* comedienne Gilda Radner who died of ovarian cancer in 1989. Membership is completely free of charge and open to men, women, and children living with cancer and their families and friends. You will find all kinds of workshops including stress reduction, meditation, yoga, etc.

....

weSPARK

www.wespark.org
Phone: (818) 906-3022
With two locations in Southern California (Sherman Oaks and Santa Clarita), weSPARK provides numerous free support groups, workshops, and classes to anyone affected by cancer.

Ginseng for Cancer-Related Fatigue

To obtain the same formulation of ginseng used by investigators at the Mayo Clinic in the pilot study of ginseng for cancer-related fatigue, contact the Ginseng Board of Wisconsin at (715) 845-7300 or at www.gingsengboard.com where you will find a link to a summary of the pilot study.

Online resources

CancerCare

www.cancercare.org
Toll free (800) 813-HOPE
CancerCare is a nonprofit organization providing free support services for anyone touched by cancer, including educational programs, fact sheets, downloadable booklets, counseling, online support groups, and help with financial assistance. They produce more than fifty one-hour telephone education workshops with

cancer experts each year and you can conference in from home or office.

....

CancerSymptoms.org

www.cancersymptoms.org

This site includes a comprehensive section about the causes and symptoms of cognitive changes and other side effects associated with cancer treatment.

....

National Coalition for Cancer Survivorship (NCCS)

www.canceradvocacy.org

Toll free: (877) NCCS-YES (1-877-622-7937)

You can reach an information specialist between 8:30 a.m. and 5:30 p.m. (EST).

The NCCS is the "oldest survivor-led cancer advocacy organization in the country," engaging in legislative advocacy for patient rights and emphasizing patient education. They also offer a free audio program called the Cancer Survival Toolbox that is intended to help people with cancer learn to communicate their needs, stand up for their rights and learn other important skills.

....

LIVESTRONG SurvivorCare Program

www.livestrong.org/survivorcare

Toll free: (866) 235-7205

Case managers available Monday-Friday from 9 a.m. to 5 p.m. (EST).

LIVESTRONG provides education, counseling services, information about treatment and side effects and help with employment, financial and insurance concerns, and more.

American Cancer Society

www.cancer.org

Toll free: (800) ACS-2345

Up-to-date information about cancer, treatment, side effects and much more.

Breastcancer.org

www.breastcancer.org

A Web site devoted to providing the latest information about breast cancer.

Clinical Trials

Before contacting investigators and to make sure the following trials (and others) are currently enrolling participants, log on at http: www.clinicaltrials.gov/ and search by key words.

David Geffen School of Medicine at UCLA, Los Angeles, California is the central site for several studies on (1) *examining the effects of cancer and cancer-therapies on cognition and brain chemistry*, and (2) *assessing the effectiveness of newly developed post-chemo rehabilitation programs*, led by investigators Daniel H. Silverman, M.D., Ph.D., and colleagues. For information about specific clinical trials ongoing at UCLA, or to check on eligibility criteria for research subjects, Dr. Silverman can be contacted via e-mail at dansilverman@ rocketmail.com.

Weill Medical College of Cornell University, New York, and **Memorial Sloan-Kettering Cancer Center, New York,** are the hosts of a study on *effects of chemotherapy and radiation therapy on cognition* *and brain structure in adult stem cell transplant recipients,* led by Dr. Denise Correa, Ph.D., and colleagues. For further information, Dr. Correa can be contacted via e-mail at corread@mskcc.org.

Memorial Sloan-Kettering Cancer Center, New York, is the site of a clinical trial on *effects of chemotherapy on changes in cognition and DNA in breast cancer survivors,* led by investigators Dr. Tim Ahles and colleagues. For more information, Dr. Ahles can be contacted via e-mail at ahlest@mskcc.org.

University Health Network, Toronto, Ontario, is the location for a study on *Cognitive Function and Fatigue in Colorectal Cancer (CRC) Patients after Chemotherapy,* led by investigators Janette Vardy, M.D., and colleagues. For information, email her at jvardy@med.usyd .edu.au.

To learn more about a **Multicenter** Phase III Randomized Study of *American Ginseng (Panax quinquefolius) in Patients With Cancer-Related Fatigue,* contact protocol co-chair Charles Loprinzi via e-mail at clo prinzi@mayo.edu.

Mayo Clinic Cancer Center in Rochester, Minnesota, is the site for a phase II randomized study of three different programs of *paced breathing in women breast cancer survivors with hot flashes.* Contact protocol chair Amit Sood, M.D., via e-mail at cancerclinicaltrials @mayo.edu.

University of Texas M.D. Anderson Cancer Center is sponsoring several mind-body studies, including: (1) *biobehavioral effects of emotional expression in (renal) cancer;* (2) *presurgical qigong therapy for women with breast cancer;* and (3) *meditation and cognitive function in women with breast cancer.* Contact principal investigator Lorenzo Cohen, Ph.D., by phone at 713-745-4260.

University of Texas M.D. Anderson Cancer Center is studying the effects of methylphenidate versus sustained release methylphenidate on cognitive functioning in patients with brain tumors. Contact principal investigator Jeffrey S. Wefel, Ph.D., at 713-792-2883.

City of Hope Comprehensive Cancer Center, Duarte, California, is the site of a study of *cognitive function in older women with stage I, stage II, or stage III breast cancer receiving hormone therapy.* Contact the Clinical Trials Office at 800-826-4673 or becomingapatient@coh.org.

Posit Science Corporation (makers of the Brain Fitness Program) in San Francisco, California, is recruiting participants for a study of computer-based training for cognitive enhancement. Contact Henry Mahncke, Ph.D., at 415-394-3100 ext. 3107 or by e-mail at henry.mahncke@positscience.com.

Books

First Things First, by Stephen R. Covey, A. Roger Merrill, and Rebecca R. Merrill (NY: Free Press, 1996).

The 7 Habits of Highly Effective People, by Stephen R. Covey (NY: Free Press, 2004).

The Memory Bible: An Innovative Strategy for Keeping Your Brain Young, by Gary Small, M.D. (NY: Hyperion, 2003). See other books by Gary Small with Gigi Vorgan.

Foods to Fight Cancer: Essential Foods to Help Prevent Cancer, by Richard Béliveau, Ph.D., and Denis Gingras, Ph.D. (New York: DK Adult, 2007).

The Omega Diet: The Lifesaving Nutritional Program Based on the Diet of the Island of Crete, by Artemis P. Simopoulos, M.D., and Jo Robinson (New York: Collins Living, 1999).

GENERIC DRUGS AND BRAND NAME EQUIVALENTS

GENERIC NAME	BRAND NAME(S)
acetaminophen plus hydrocodone	Vicodin
acetaminophen plus oxycodone	Percocet, Roxicet
anastrozole	Arimidex
carboplatin	Paraplatin, Novaplus
carmustine	BiCNU, Gliadel
cisplatin	Platinol
cyclophosphamide	Cytoxan and Neosar
cytarabine	Cytosar, Tarabine, Cytosar
dacarbazine	DTIC-Dome
darbepoetin alfa	Aranesp
dexmethylphenidate	Focalin
docetaxel	Taxotere
doxorubicin	Adriamycin, Doxil, Evacet, Rubex
etoposide	VePesid, VP-16, Etopophos, Toposar
exemestane	Aromasin
fulvestrant	Faslodex
gemcitabine	Gemzar
idarubicin	Idamycin, Zavedos
letrozole	Femara
lorazepam	Ativan
melphalan	Alkeran
methotrexate	Rheumatrex, Trexall, Folex
modafinil	Provigil
paclitaxel	Taxol, Onxol
pegfilgrastim	Neulasta
raloxifene	Evista
rituximab	Rituxan

CONTINUES

Generic Drugs and Brand Name Equivalents

GENERIC NAME	BRAND NAME(S)
topotecan	Hycamtin
toremifene	Fareston
trastuzumab	Herceptin
vinblastine	Velban
vincristine	Oncovin, Vincasar, Marqibo
warfarin	Coumadin, Jantoven

Notes

Chapter 1

1 Diagnostic and Statistical Manual of Mental Disorders, fourth edition, 309.81 Posttraumatic Stress Disorder accessed at http:www.psychiatryonline.com/content.aspx?aID=3357&search-Str=post-traumatic+stress+disorder.

2 M. Gurevich, et al., "Psychosomatics Stress Response Syndromes and Cancer: Conceptual and Assessment Issues," *Psychosomatics* 43 (2002): 259–281. Accessed at http:psy.psychiatryonline.org/cgi/content/full/43/4/259.

3 Find survey results at http:www.hurricanevoices.org.

Chapter 2

1 A. Hurria, et al., "Renaming 'Chemobrain,'" *Cancer Investigation* 25 (2007): 373–377.

2 J. Wefel, et al., "The Cognitive Sequelae of Standard-Dose Adjuvant Chemotherapy in Women with Breast Carcinoma," *Cancer* 100, no. 11 (2004): 2292–2299.

3 A. Hurria, et al., "Cognitive Function of Older Patients Receiving Adjuvant Chemotherapy for Breast Cancer: A Pilot Prospective Longitudinal Study," *Journal of the American Geriatrics Society* 54, no. 6 (2006): 925–931.

Chapter 3

1 J. L. Zeller, "Cancer Chemotherapy," *Journal of the American Medical Association* (JAMA) 299, no. 22 (2008): 2706.

2 American Medical Association, Informed Consent, accessed at http:www.ama-assn.org/ama/pub/category/4608.html.

3 R. Ferguson and T. Ahles, "Low Neuropsychologic Performance Among Adult Cancer Survivors Treated with Chemotherapy," *Current Neurology & Neuroscience Reports* 3, no. 3 (2003): 215–222.

4 D. H. Silverman, et al., "Altered Frontocortical, Cerebellar, and Basal Ganglia Activity in Adjuvant-Treated Breast Cancer Survivors 5–10 Years After Chemotherapy," *Breast Cancer Research and Treatment* 103, no. 3 (Epub 2006): 303–311; F. S. van Dam, et al., "Impairment of Cognitive Function in Women Receiving Adjuvant Treatment for High-Risk Breast Cancer: High-Dose Versus Standard-Dose Chemotherapy," *Journal of the National Cancer Institute* (JNCI) 90 (1998): 210–218. Accessed at http: jnci.oxfordjournals.org/cgi/reprint/90/3/210.

5 Early Breast Cancer Trialists' Collaborative Group (EBCTCG), "Effects of Chemotherapy and Hormonal Therapy for Early Breast Cancer on Recurrence and 15-Year Survival: An Overview of the Randomized Trials," *Lancet* 365 (2005): 1687–1717.

6 Accessed at http:www.breastcancer.org/treatment/hormonal/ what_is_it/hormone_role.jsp.

7 T. Ahles, A. Saykin, et al., "The Relationship of APOE Genotype to Neuropsychological Performance in Long-Term Cancer Survivors Treated with Standard Dose Chemotherapy," *Psycho-Oncology* 12, no. 6 (2003): 612–619.

8 American Cancer Society Facts & Figures 2008,

9 H. Muss, et al., "Toxicity of Older and Younger Patients Treated With Adjuvant Chemotherapy for Node-Positive Breast Cancer: The Cancer and Leukemia Group B Experience," *Journal of Clinical Oncology* 25, no. 24 (2007): 3699–3704.

10 M. Pinder, et al., "Congestive Heart Failure in Older Women Treated With Adjuvant Anthracycline Chemotherapy for Breast Cancer." *Journal of Clinical Oncology* 25, no. 25 (2007): 3808–3815.

11 T. Fried, et al., "Understanding the Treatment Preferences of Seriously Ill Patients," *New England Journal of Medicine* 346, no. 14 (2002): 1061–1066.

Chapter 6

1 R. Brown and D. McNeill, "The 'Tip of the Tongue' Phenomenon," *Journal of Verbal Learning and Verbal Behavior* 5 (1966): 325–337.

2 F. Downie, et al., "Cognitive Function, Fatigue, and Menopausal Symptoms in Breast Cancer Patients Receiving Adjuvant Chemotherapy: Evaluation with Patient Interview after Formal Assessment," *Psycho-Oncology* 15 (2006): 921–930.

Chapter 7

1 National Comprehensive Cancer Network, "Cancer-Related Fatigue and Anemia: Treatment Guidelines for Patients,"

(2005). Accessed at http:www.nccn.org/patients/patient_gls/_english/pdf/NCCN%20Fatigue%20Guidelines.pdf.

2 N. de Jong, et al., "Course of Mental Fatigue and Motivation in Breast Cancer Patients Receiving Adjuvant Chemotherapy," *Annals of Oncology* 16, no. 3 (2005): 372–382.

3 N. de Jong, et al., "Prevalence and Course of Fatigue in Breast Cancer Patients Receiving Adjuvant Chemotherapy." *Annals of Oncology* 15 (2004): 896–905.

4 Accessed at http:www.cancer.org/docroot/MIT/content/MIT_2_4X_Depression.asp and NIH Publication No. 03–5121, 65. Accessed January 2003 at http:www.nimh.nih.gov/about/strategic-planning-reports/breaking-ground-breaking-through—the-strategic-plan-for-mood-disorders-research.pdf.

5 American Psychiatric Association, *Diagnostic and Statistical Manual of Mental Disorders*, fourth edition (DSM-IV).

Chapter 8

1 Adapted, from Christina A. Meyers, Ph.D., University of Texas MD Anderson Cancer Center.

Chapter 9

1 J. Wefel, et al., "The Cognitive Sequelae of Standard-Dose Adjuvant Chemotherapy in Women with Breast Carcinoma: Results of a Prospective, Randomized, Longitudinal Trial," *Cancer* 100 (2004): 2292–2299.

2 C. Bender, et al., "Cognitive Impairment Associated with Adjuvant Therapy in Breast Cancer," *Psycho-Oncology* 15 (2006): 422–430.

3 A. Hurria, et al. "Cognitive Function of Older Patients Receiving Adjuvant Chemotherapy for Breast Cancer: A Pilot Prospective

Longitudinal Study," *Journal of the American Geriatric Society* 54 (2006): 925–931.

4 H. Fan, et al., "Fatigue, Menopausal Symptoms, and Cognitive Function in Women after Adjuvant Chemotherapy for Breast Cancer: 1- and 2-Year Follow-Up of a Prospective Controlled Study," *Journal of Clinical Oncology* 23 (2005): 8025–8032.

5 S. Schagen, et al., "Change in Cognitive Function after Chemotherapy: A Prospective Longitudinal Study in Breast Cancer Patients," *Journal of the National Cancer Institute* 98 (2006): 1742–1745.

6 V. Jenkins, et al., "A 3-Year Prospective Study of the Effects of Adjuvant Treatments on Cognition in Women with Early Stage Breast Cancer," *British Journal of Cancer* 94 (2006): 828–834.

7 C. Quesnel, et al., "Cognitive Impairments Associated with Breast Cancer Treatments: Results from a Longitudinal Study," *Breast Cancer Research and Treatment* (2008).

8 C. Jansen, et al., "Preliminary Results of a Longitudinal Study of Changes in Cognitive Function in Breast Cancer Patients Undergoing Chemotherapy with Doxorubicin and Cyclophosphamide," *Psycho-Oncology* (2008).

9 A. Stewart, et al., "The Cognitive Effects of Adjuvant Chemotherapy in Early Stage Breast Cancer: A Prospective Study," *Psycho-Oncology* (2008): 122–130.

Chapter 10

1 When Einstein died in 1955, a pathologist at Princeton Hospital removed Einstein's brain and cut the cerebral hemispheres into about 240 blocks. He stored the brain for years at his home—but that is another tale.

2 S. F. Witelson, et al., "The Exceptional Brain of Albert Einstein" *Lancet* 353, no. 9170 (1999): 2149–2153.

Chapter 11

1 B. Kreukels and S. Schagen, et al., "Electrophysiological Correlates of Information Processing in Breast Cancer Patients Treated with Adjuvant Chemotherapy," *Breast Cancer Research and Treatment* 94, no. 1 (2005): 53–61. Abstract accessed online at http:www.springerlink.com/content/k122168q55u20013.

2 J. Dietrich and R. Han, et al., "CNS Progenitor Cells and Oligodendrocytes Are Targets of Chemotherapeutic Agents In Vitro and In Vivo," *Journal of Biology* 5:22 (2006). Accessed online at http: jbiol.com/content/pdf/jbiol5.pdf.

3 G. Winocur, "The Effects of the Anti-Cancer Drugs Methotrexate and 5-Fluorouracil on Cognitive Function in Mice," *Pharmacology Biochemistry and Behavior* 85, no. 1 (2006): 66–75. Abstract accessed online at http:www.scopus.com/scopus/record/display.url?eid=2-s2.0–33751307914&view=basic&origin=inward&txGid=gyx5KL2_ztDStzimKqvsT4l%3a2.

4 M. Inagaki, et al. "Smaller Regional Volumes of Brain Gray and White Matter Demonstrated in Breast Cancer Survivors Exposed to Adjuvant Chemotherapy," *Cancer* 109, no. 1 (2006): 146–156. Abstract accessed online at http:www3.interscience.wiley.com/cgi-bin/abstract/113489209/ABSTRACT.

5 D. H. Silverman, et al., "Altered Frontocortical, Cerebellar, and Basal Ganglia Activity in Adjuvant-Treated Breast Cancer Survivors 5–10 Years After Chemotherapy," *Breast Cancer Research and Treatment* 103, no. 3 (2006): 303–311. Abstract accessed online at http:www.springerlink.com/content/mq53511v473 u2253/.

6 A. Gangloff, et al. "Estimation of Paclitaxel Biodistribution and

Uptake in Human-Derived Xenografts In Vivo with 18F-Fluoropaclitaxel," *The Journal of Nuclear Medicine* 46, no. 11 (2005): 1866–1871. Accessed online at http:jnm.snmjournals.org/cgi/reprint/46/11/1866.pdf.

Chapter 12

1 A. Minisini, et al., "What Is the Effect of Systemic Anticancer Treatment on Cognitive Function?" *Lancet Oncology* 5, no. 5 (2004): 273–282.

2 Sandra Blakeslee, "Female Sex Hormone Is Tied to Ability to Perform Tasks," *New York Times*, Nov. 18, 1988. Accessed online at http:query.nytimes.com/gst/fullpage.html?res=940DE5D 91239F93BA25752C1A96E948260.

3 E. Hampson and D. Kimura, "Reciprocal Effects of Hormonal Fluctuations on Human Motor and Perceptual-Spatial Skills," *Behavioral Neuroscience* 102, No. 3 (1988): 456–459; and E. Hampson, "Spatial Cognition in Humans: Possible Modulation by Androgens and Estrogens." *Psychiatry Neuroscience* 20, no. 5 (1995): 397–404.

4 B. Sherwin and T. Tulandi, "'Add-Back' Estrogen Reverses Cognitive Deficits Induced by a Gonadotropin-Releasing Hormone Agonist in Women with Leiomyomata Uteri," *Journal of Clinical Endocrinology and Metabolism* 81, no. 7: 2545–2549.

5 Early Breast Cancer Trialists' Collaborative Group, "Tamoxifen for Early Breast Cancer: An Overview of the Randomized Trials," *Lancet* 351 (1998): 1451–1467.

6 C. Bender, et al., "Cognitive Impairment Associated with Adjuvant Therapy in Breast Cancer," *Psycho-Oncology* 15, no. 5 (2006): 422–430. Abstract accessed online at http:www3.interscience.wiley.com/journal/110579669/abstract

7   The ATAC Trialists Group, "Pharmacokinetics of Anastrozole and Tamoxifen Alone, and in Combination, During Adjuvant Endocrine Therapy for Early Breast Cancer in Postmenopausal Women: A Sub-Protocol of the 'Arimidex and Tamoxifen Alone or in Combination' (ATAC) Trial," *British Journal of Cancer* 85 (2001): 317–324.

8   C. Bender, et al. "Memory Impairments with Adjuvant Anastrozole Versus Tamoxifen in Women with Early-Stage Breast Cancer," *Menopause* 14, no. 6 (2007): 995–998.

9   N. L. Rasgon, ed., Estrogen's Effects in the Central Nervous System: Estrogen and Mood. Estrogen's Effects on Brain Function— What's Next? (Baltimore, MD: John Hopkins Press, 2006).

10 National Cancer Institute, accessed online at http:www.cancer. gov/clinicaltrials/results/gabapentin-meno607.

11 C. L. Loprinzi, et al., "Venlafaxine in Management of Hot Flashes in Survivors of Breast Cancer: A Randomized Controlled Trial," *Lancet* 356 (2000): 2059–2063.

12 P. Maki, et al., "Objective Hot Flashes Are Negatively Related to Verbal Memory Performance in Midlife Women," *Menopause* 15, no. 5 (2008).

13 The Women's Health Initiative, http:www.nhlbi.nih.gov/whi.

14 National Cancer Institute, http:www.cancer.gov/clinicaltrials/ digest-postmenopausal-hormone-use.

15 Women's Health Initiative Memory Study, http:www1.wfub mc.edu/whims.

16 Women's Health Initiative, Estrogen-Alone Study, http: www.nhlbi.nih.gov/whi/estro_alone.htm.

17 S. Shumaker, et al., "Estrogen Plus Progestin and the Incidence of Dementia and Mild Cognitive Impairment in Postmenopausal

Women" (The Women's Health Initiative Memory Study: A Randomized Controlled Trial), *The Journal of the American Medical Association* (JAMA) 289, no. (2003): 2651–2662. Abstract accessed online at http:jama.ama-assn.org/cgi/content/abstract/289/20/2651.

18 J. Manson, et al., "Estrogen Therapy and Coronary-Artery Calcification," *New England Journal of Medicine* (NEJM) 356 (2007): 2591–2602.

19 N. Krieger, et al., "Hormone Replacement Therapy, Cancer, Controversies, and Women's Health: Historical, Epidemiological, Biological, Clinical, and Advocacy Perspectives," *Journal of Epidemiology and Community Health* 59 (2005): 740–748.

20 E. Salminen, et al., "Estradiol and Cognition During Androgen Deprivation in Men with Prostate Carcinoma," *Cancer* 103, no. 7 (2005): 1381–1387.

21 M. Cherrier, et. al., "The Role of Aromatization in Testosterone Supplementation: Effects on Cognition in Older Men," *Neurology* 64 (2005): 290–296.

22 World Health Organization and American Cancer Society.

23 American Cancer Society, Detailed Guide: What Are the Key Statistics About Prostate Cancer? Accessed online at http: www.cancer.org.

24 F. Joly, et al., "Impact of Androgen Deprivation Therapy on Physical and Cognitive Function, As Well As Quality of Life of Patients with Nonmetastatic Prostate Cancer," *Journal of Urology* 176, no. 6 (2006): 2443–2447.

Chapter 13

1 Accessed online at http:www.cancer.org/docroot/MIT/con-

tent/MIT_2_4X_Depression.asp and NIH Publication No. 03–5121, p. 65, January 2003, accessed online at http:www.nimh .nih.gov/about/strategic-planning-reports/breaking-ground-breaking-through—the-strategic-plan-for-mood-disorders-research .pdf.

2 P.A. Lewis, et al., "Brain Mechanisms for Mood Congruent Memory Facilitation," *NeuroImage* 25, no. 4 (2005): 1214–1223.

3 Accessed online at http:www.fda.gov/cder/drug/InfoSheets/patient/FluoxetinePIS.pdf.

4 Accessed online at http:www.cfsan.fda.gov/~dms/ds-take.html #risks.

5 T. Klassen, et al., "Mood Congruent Memory Bias Induced by Tryptophan Depletion," *Psychological Medicine* 32 (2002): 167–172.

6 Accessed online at http:lpi.oregonstate.edu/infocenter/othernuts/choline.

Chapter 14

1 Accessed online at http:www.cancer.gov/cancertopics/pdq/ supportivecare/sleepdisorders.

2 A. Williamson and A. Feyer, " Moderate Sleep Deprivation Produces Impairments in Cognitive and Motor Performance Equivalent to Legally Prescribed Levels of Alcohol Intoxication," *Occupational and Environmental Medicine* 57 (2000): 649–655.

3 Sources: Sweden, Australia, Belgium, Greece, Canada, UK: The World Health Organization, *World Report on Road Traffic Injury Report* (2004), accessed online at www.who.int/violence_injury_prevention/en/; United States: NHTSA, http:www-nrd.nhtsa.dot.gov/Pubs/810801.PDF, updated March 2008.

4 J. Ellenbogen, et al., "Human Relational Memory Requires Time and Sleep," The National Academy of Sciences, *PNAS* 104, no.

18 (2007): 7723–7728.

5 S. C. Mednick, et al., "The Restorative Effect of Naps on Perceptual Deterioration," *Nature Neuroscience* 5 (2002): 677–681.

6 E. Schernhammer and S. Hankinson, "Urinary Melatonin Levels and Breast Cancer Risk," *Journal of the National Cancer Institute* 97 (2005): 1084–1087.

7 E. Schernhammer, et al., "Night-Shift Work and Risk of Colorectal Cancer in the Nurses' Health Study," *Journal of the National Cancer Institute* 95 (2003): 825–828.

Chapter 15

1 F. Baker, et al. "Adult Cancer Survivors: How Are They Faring?" *Cancer* (supplement) 104, no. 11 (2005): 2565–2576. See article online at http:www3.interscience.wiley.com/cgi-bin/fulltext/112134333/PDFSTART.

2 B. Cimprich and D. Ronis, "An Environmental Intervention to Restore Attention in Women With Newly Diagnosed Breast Cancer," *Cancer Nursing* 26, no. 4 (2003): 284–292.

3 S. Kaplan, "Meditation, Restoration, and the Management of Mental Fatigue," *Environment and Behavior* 33, no. 4 (2001): 480–506.

4 Accessed online at http:www.cspinet.org/new/cafchart.htm.

5 A note about government oversight of dietary supplements: The FDA has recently instituted a new rule called *Final Rule* that regulates the quality, content, and manufacturing processes of dietary supplements, although the FDA does not test supplements prior to manufacturing. Manufacturers will now be required to substantiate the safety of their products and provide evidence that representations or claims made about their products are not false or misleading. The FDA required large man-

ufacturers to comply by June 2008. Smaller companies will phase in controls through June 2010. Source: FDA Fact Sheet, Dietary Supplement Current Good Manufacturing Practices and Interim Final Rule Facts, http:www.cfsan.fda.gov/~dms/dscgmps6.html.

Chapter 16

1 P. Sarkar, et al., "Ontogeny of Foetal Exposure to Maternal Cortisol Using Midtrimester Amniotic Fluid As a Biomarker," *Clinical Endocrinology* 66, no. 5 (2007): 636–640.

2 K. Bergman, et al., "Maternal Stress During Pregnancy Predicts Cognitive Ability and Fearfulness in Infancy," *Journal of the American Academy of Child & Adolescent Psychiatry* 46, no. 11 (2007): 1454–1463.

3 M. F. Johnston, et al., "Acupuncture for Chemotherapy-Associated Cognitive Dysfunction: A Hypothesis-Generating Literature Review to Inform Clinical Advice," *Integrative Cancer Therapies* 6, no. 1 (2007): 36–41.

4 J. Bower, et al., "Yoga for Cancer Patients and Survivors," *Cancer Control* 12, no. 3 (2005):165–171. Accessed online at http:www.moffitt.org/moffittapps/ccjv12n3/pdf/165.pdf.

5 L. Cohen, et al., "Psychological Adjustment and Sleep Quality in a Randomized Trial of the Effects of a Tibetan Yoga Intervention in Patients with Lymphoma," *Cancer* 100, no. 10 (2004): 2253–2260.

6 R. J. Davidson, et al., "Long-Term Meditators Self-Induce High Amplitude Gamma Synchrony During Mental Practice," The National Academy of Sciences, *PNAS* 101, no. 46 (2004): 16369–16373.

7 The scientists used magnetic resonance imaging to record the

thickness of the cortex—the outer area of the brain—in twenty people who had an average of nine years of meditation experience and practiced six hours per week. A control group of fifteen individuals had no meditation or yoga experience. S. W. Lazar, et al., "Meditation Experience Is Associated with Increased Cortical Thickness," *NeuroReport* 16, no. 17 (2005): 1893–1897.

Chapter 17

1 "California Bars Restaurant Use of Trans Fats," *New York Times*, July 26, 2008. Accessed online at http:www.nytimes.com/2008/07/26/us/26fats.html?ref=health.

2 Food and Drug Administration, accessed online at http: www.cfsan.fda.gov/~dms/qatrans2.html#s1q3.

3 Artemis P. Simopoulos, M.D., and Jo Robinson, *The Omega Diet: The Lifesaving Nutritional Program Based on the Diet of the Island of Crete* (New York: Harper Perennial, 1999).

4 F. Calon, et al., "Docosahexaenoic Acid Protects From Dendritic Pathology in an Alzheimer's Disease Mouse Model," *Neuron* 43, no. 5 (2004): 633–645.

5 G. Fontani, et al., "Cognitive and Physiological Effects of Omega-3 Polyunsaturated Fatty Acid Supplementation in Healthy Subjects," *European Journal of Clinical Investigation* 35 (2005): 691–699.

6 Ronald A. Hites, et al., "Global Assessment of Organic Contaminants in Farmed Salmon," *Science* 303 (2004): 226–229. Abstract: http:www.sciencemag.org/cgi/content/abstract/303/5655/226

7 A. P. Simopoulos, "Genetics and Nutrition: Or What Your Genes Can Tell You About Nutrition," *World Review of Nutrition and Dietetics* 63 (1990): 25–34.

8 U.S. Department of Agriculture, Nutrient Data Laboratory.

9 Linus Pauling Institute, accessed online at http:lpi.oregonstate .edu/infocenter/phytochemicals/carotenoids/index.html.

10 Neal Barnard, *The Survivor's Handbook: Eating Right for Cancer Survival* (Washington, DC: The Cancer Project, 2004).

11 T. Satoh, et al., "Carnosic Acid, A Catechol-Type Electrophilic Compound, Protects Neurons Both In Vitro and In Vivo . . . ," *Journal of Neurochemistry* 104, no. 4 (2008): 1116–1131.

12 C. F. Garland, et al., "The Role of Vitamin D in Cancer Prevention," *American Journal of Public Health* 96, no. 2 (2006):252-261; and M. F. Holick, "The Vitamin D Epidemic and Its Health Consequences," *Journal of Nutrition* 135 (2005): 2739S–2748S.

13 Ibid.

14 Accessed online at http:ods.od.nih.gov/factsheets/vitamind .asp.

15 Accessed online at http:lpi.oregonstate.edu/infocenter/vitamins/vitaminB12/index.html#food_source.

16 K. Conklin, "Coenzyme Q10 for Prevention of Anthracycline-Induced Cardiotoxicity," *Integrative Cancer Therapies* 4, no. 2 (2005): 110–130 (2005). Abstract accessed online at http:ict .sagepub.com/cgi/content/abstract/4/2/110.

17 C. Shults, et al., "Effects of Coenzyme Q10 in Early Parkinson Disease: Evidence of Slowing of the Functional Decline," *Archives of Neurology* 59, no. 10 (2002): 1541–1550.

18 Linus Pauling Institute, accessed online at http:lpi.oregonstate. edu/infocenter/othernuts/coq10/.

19 A. Heck, et al., "Potential Interactions Between Alternative Therapies and Warfarin," *American Journal of Health-System Pharmacy* 57 (2000): 1221–1227.

20 S. T. DeKosky, et al., "Ginkgo Biloba for Prevention of Dementia:

A Randomized Controlled Trial," *JAMA* 300, no. 19 (2008): 2253–2262. Accessed online at http:jama.ama-assn.org/cgi/ content/ full/300/19/.

Chapter 18

1 Y. Hirano, et al., "Effects of Chewing in Working Memory Processing," *Neuroscience Letters* 436 (2008): 189–192.

Chapter 19

1 *American Journal of Medicine* 121 (2008):551–552.

2 R. F. Riemersma-van der Lek, et al., "Effect of Bright Light and Melatonin on Cognitive and Noncognitive Function in Elderly Residents of Group Care Facilities: A Randomized Controlled Trial," *Journal of the American Medical Association (JAMA)* 299 (2008): 2642–2655.

3 Adapted from multiple internally corroborated sources; most comprehensive is the "USDA National Nutrient Database for Standard Reference, Release 18, Protein (g) Content of Selected Foods per Common Measure," available at URL www.nal.us da.gov/fnic/foodcomp/Data/SR18/nutrlist/sr18a203.pdf

4 Tjonneland, et al., "Alcohol Intake and Breast Cancer Risk: The European Prospective Investigation into Cancer and Nutrition (EPIC)," *Cancer Causes and Control* 18, no. 4 (2007): 361–373.

5 M. Groenbaek, et al., "Type of Alcohol Consumed and Mortality From All Causes, Coronary Heart Disease, and Cancer," *Annals of Internal Medicine* 133 (2000): 411–419.

6 K. Mehlig, et al., "Alcoholic Beverages and Incidence of Dementia," *American Journal of Epidemiology* 167 (2008): 684–691.

7 R. A. Emmons and M. E. McCullough, "Counting Blessings

Versus Burdens: Experimental Studies of Gratitude and Subjective Well-Being in Daily Life," *Journal of Personality and Social Psychology* 84 (2003): 377–389.

8 When you *really need* professional advice or medical care, by all means get it.

Chapter 21

1 A. Minisini, et al., "What Is the Effect of Systemic Anticancer Treatment on Cognitive Function?" *Lancet, Oncology* 5 (2004): 273–282.

2 Idelle Davidson interview with Ian Tannock, M.D., Ph.D., February 7, 2008.

3 Accessed online at University of Auckland, pharmacology http:intro.phm.auckland.ac.nz/lectures%202007/Lecture%202%20-%20What%20is%20a%20Drug.pdf.

4 L. Tsai, et al., "Recovery of Learning and Memory Is Associated with Chromatin Remodeling," *Nature* 447 (2007): 178–183.

5 Press release from Howard Hughes Medical Institute, April 29, 2007, "Enhanced Environment Restores Memory in Mice with Neurodegeneration." Accessed online at http:www. hhmi.org/news/tsai20070429.html.

Index

Acetylcholine, 127, 132
Acupuncture, 166
Adenosine triphosphate (ATP), 183, 189
Adrenaline, 157, 206, 208
    See also Epinephrine
Adriamycin, 16
Ahles, Tim, 6, 21
Alcohol, 212–215, 223
Alpert, Joe, 202–203, 204, 219
Alpha-linolenic acid, 176
Alzheimer's disease, xvi, 64, 66, 114
    and brain imaging, 229
    and chemo brain, 20–21
    and drugs, 97, 100, 127
    and exercise, 164
    and fatty acids, 177–178
    and ginkgo biloba, 190
    and recovering memories, 235, 236, 237

ruling out, 68–69
American Cancer Society, 10, 143
American Heart Association, 211
American Journal of Medicine, 202
American Psychiatric Association, 3
Anastrozole, 17, 107, 108
Androgens, 116–117
Anemia, 8, 56–57
Anesthesia, 8, 11
Annals of Internal Medicine, 214
Anthracycline drugs, 16, 23
    See also particular anthracyclines
Antihormonal therapies, 9, 11, 15, 106–108, 117, 231
    See also Hormonal therapy;
    Tamoxifen
Antioxidants, 183–190, 207, 209, 211, 212, 222
Anxiety
    and acupuncture, 166
    and alcohol, 212

and bupropion, 129
and cancer, 8, 59–60, 156, 161, 162
and chemotherapy, 21, 55, 75
and cognitive therapy, 123
and depression, 128, 156
drugs for treating, 130–131, 140
and fear, 59–60
and GABA, 127
and ginseng, 148
and insomnia, 134, 135, 139
and learned helplessness, 205
and meditation, 170
and omega-3 fatty acids, 178
and perceived cognitive
    impairment, 64
and serotonin, 126
and visits with oncologists, xvi, 13
ApoE4, 20–21
Aromatase inhibitors, 17, 106–108,
    110
Attention, 70
    and brain, 83, 125, 170
    and caffeine, 147
    and chemotherapy, 10, 25, 49–50,
        62, 67, 69, 72
    and chemotherapy: and fatigue
        and depression, 55, 57, 58, 121,
        144, 145
    and Kaplan's restoration theory,
        145–147
    and meditation, 169, 170
    and memory, 49, 50, 51, 62, 69
    and nature, 144–145, 146–147
    and stimulants, 130, 150, 153
    training, 48, 195
Attention deficit disorder (ADD), 40,
    150
Attention deficit hyperactivity disor-
    der (ADHD), 11, 153

Barton, Debra, 148–150
Behavior modification techniques,
    164

Bender, Catherine, 107, 108
Benzodiazepines (BZs), 130–131, 140
Beta-carotene, 184–185
Biological clock, 206–207, 223
Bladder cancer, 32
Bone marrow transplants, 56
Brain
    and acupuncture, 166
    and alcohol, 212
    and Alzheimer's, 20
    basal ganglia, 52, 231
    blood-brain barrier, 93–94, 96, 116,
        226–227, 228, 229
    and caffeine, 211
    cancer, 230
    cerebellum, 52, 82, 85
    cerebral cortex, 80, 81, 170, 196
    cerebrum, 82, 83, 84, 85
    changes and chemotherapy, viii,
        20, 66, 86–98, 227, 228, 229
    and coenzyme Q10, 189
    and cognitive reserve hypothesis,
        22
    and compensating for
        impairments, 96–97
    and depression, 24, 121, 124–129
    diagram of regions and their roles,
        82
    and executive functioning, 45, 46,
        84, 97, 103
    exercising, 70, 98, 194, 217
    and fats, 172–174, 177–178, 190
    and free radicals, 183, 184
    frontal lobes, 80, 82, 83–84
    "Games," 195
    and genes, 205
    and ginkgo biloba, 189
    and gum chewing, 196
    healthy, 79–85
    and hormones, 100, 101, 103, 105,
        114, 115–116, 141
    hypothalamus, nucleus
        accumbens, amygdala, and hip-

pocampus, 84–85, 103, 105, 111, 158, 164, 196, 216

imaging, 228–231, 235 (see also Brain: PET scans)

injury and worsening personal characteristics, 68

and language, 47, 83, 86, 89, 92

limbic system, 79–80

and meditation, 169–170

and memory, 45, 52, 80, 81, 82, 83–84, 85, 89, 90, 91, 92, 97, 103, 105, 116, 121, 125, 158, 164, 196, 235, 236

and milk, 211

and natural environment, 146–147

neurons and neurotransmitters, 80–81, 86–87, 92, 97, 99–100, 124–129, 131, 132, 164, 206, 207, 208, 211, 221–222, 229, 236

and neuroplasticity, 169–170

occipital, parietal, and temporal lobes, 81, 82, 83, 85, 105

PET scans, 22, 24, 25–27, 89, 91, 92–93, 94, 97, 105, 114, 229–231, 234

and physical exercise, 164, 215

and phytochemicals, 186

R-complex, 79

repairing damaged chemistry of, 201–220, 221–224

and sleep, 136–137, 138, 206–207

stem, 79, 82, 84, 126

and stress, 157–158

triune, 79

unhealthy, 86–98

See also Chemo brain

Brain function

and chemotherapy, 4–7, 12, 97 (see also Brain: changes and chemotherapy; Chemo brain; Cognitive problems: and chemotherapy)

and diet, 211

and fats, 174, 178

and hormones, 105

improving, 118

and measuring forgetfulness, 62

and PET scans and other imaging, 26, 92–93, 229, 230

and sleep, 136

BRCA 1 gene, 102

Breast cancer, 37

and age, 10, 23, 32

and alcohol, 212–215

and anthracyclines, 16, 23

and chemotherapy, x, xi, xii, xv, 9–10, 11–12, 16, 17, 18, 23, 24, 51

and chemotherapy: and brain injury, 66, 87, 88–90, 91, 94, 95, 226

and chemotherapy: and cognitive domains, 45, 46, 47, 48–49

and chemotherapy: and fatigue and depression, 57–58, 152

and chemotherapy: and hormones and menopause, 99, 101, 102–103, 107, 110, 117

and chemotherapy: and measuring forgetfulness, 61

and chemotherapy: and sensitivity testing, 233–234

and chemotherapy: and strategies for dealing with effects, 192, 197

and chemotherapy: studies, 72–73, 74–75, 88–90

and CMF, 16, 58

of coauthor, ix–xvii

and cyclophosphamide, 16, 58, 74

and endocrine therapy, 63–64

and Herceptin and HER-2, x–xi, xv

and hot flashes, 112

and Hurricane Voices, 4, 5

and LaRue, 108–111

and melatonin, 141

and modafinil, 151

and nature, 144–145

and paclitaxel, 235
and PET scans, 93, 230
and post-chemo survivors, 32
and tamoxifen and other hormonal
    therapies, 17, 18, 72, 75, 89, 90,
    106–108, 110, 113
and Vitamin D, 187
and yoga, 167–168
See also Radiation: and breast
    cancer
Bupropion, 129, 216
Buspirone, 131

Caffeine, 147–148, 209, 211
Calcitriol, 187
Cancer
    and age, 10, 22–23
    and alcohol, 212–215
    and clinical depression, 58–59, 122
    and drugs derived from plants, 235
    and fear, 59–60, 156, 161, 162–163,
        167
    and future treatments, 225
    and stress, 3, 14, 145–146, 156
    support groups, xiv, xv, 6, 53, 123,
        157, 218, 219 (see also Gilda's
        Club; Wellness Community)
    See also specific cancers
Carmustine, 87, 88
Carnegie, Dale, 218
Castellon, Steven, 63–66, 67–69, 70,
    71
Center for Science in the Public
    Interest, 147
Chemo brain, 19, 100
    and Alzheimer's, 20–21, 69
    and changes in brain, viii, 20, 86,
        87, 90, 96–97, 97–98, 228
    of coauthor, x, xv–xvii
    convincing oneself of, 64
    and cyclophosphamide, 16
    and cytokines, 228
    and dementia, 21–22

and depression, 121
and family, 34
and FDA approval of drugs, 234
and hormonal therapies, 17
imprecision of, 8–9
and memory, 25, 50, 52, 53, 54,
    237
other factors in, 8
repairing damaged chemistry of,
    201–220, 221–224 ·
and research, xvii, 71–75, 86, 87
and scans, 91–92, 93
strategies for dealing with, 191–197
and types of people, 19–20
workshop on, 6
Chemosensitivity testing, 232–234
Chemotherapy
    and Alzheimer's, dementia, and
        age, 20–24
    and ApoE4, 21
    designer, 231–234
    determining whether to undergo,
        13–27
    and healthy cells, 56, 94, 97, 233
        (see also Brain: changes and
        chemotherapy)
    and oral drugs, 22
    and relationships and family, 34,
        36, 38–43
    and side effects (see Attention: and
        chemotherapy; Brain: changes
        and chemotherapy; Brain func-
        tion: and chemotherapy; Chemo
        brain; Cognitive problems: and
        chemotherapy; Concentration:
        and chemotherapy; Depression:
        and chemotherapy; Fatigue: and
        chemotherapy; Fogginess; Hair
        loss; Hormones: and chemo-
        therapy; Language: and
        chemotherapy; Learning: and
        chemotherapy; Loss of self;
        Memory: and chemotherapy;

Multitasking; Nausea; Organization)
and survival, 18, 23
See also Breast cancer: and chemotherapy; Estrogen: and chemotherapy; Menopause: and chemotherapy
Chemotherapy-induced cognitive impairment, xvii
Cholesterol, 172, 178, 183
Choline, 132, 183
Cholinesterase inhibitors, 97
Cimprich, Bernadine, 146–147
Cisplatin, 16, 40, 87, 88
Coenzyme Q10, 188–189
Cognitive distortions, 162–163
Cognitive problems
    and chemotherapy, vii–viii, 4–7, 9–12, 14–17, 100
    and chemotherapy: and Alzheimer's, dementia, and age, 20–24
    and chemotherapy: and cognitive domains, 44–54
    and chemotherapy: and fatigue, depression, and anxiety, 55–60, 63, 121
    and chemotherapy: and hormones and menopause, 101–103, 107, 110, 111–112, 117
    and chemotherapy: and rehabilitation, 201–220, 221–224
    and chemotherapy: measuring problems, 61–70
    and chemotherapy: monitoring problems, 25–27
    and chemotherapy: online survey of symptoms, 31–34
    and chemotherapy: Patrick's story, 35–37
    and chemotherapy: percentages of people, 5, 10, 19, 63, 72, 73, 74
    and chemotherapy: sorting out

causation, 225–228
    and chemotherapy: strategies for dealing with, 191–197
    and chemotherapy: studies on, 71–75
    and chemotherapy: symptom trends, 19, 20, 33, 63, 71–75, 89
    and other factors, 8
    See also Chemo brain; specific cognitive problems
Cognitive reserve hypothesis, 22
Cognitive therapy, 123–124, 218
Colantuono, Janet, 4–5, 31–33
Colon cancer, xvi, 22, 32, 113, 141, 187, 230
Combined reuptake inhibitors and receptor blockers, 130
Concentration
    and attention, 50
    and caffeine, 147
    and cancer career, 60
    and chemotherapy, xvi, 4, 25, 33, 39, 50, 67, 89, 91, 226, 228
    and chemotherapy: and fatigue and depression, 55, 56, 58, 59, 63, 121, 122, 144
    and drugs, 130, 131, 150, 151
    and gum chewing, 196
    and memory, 62
    and scans, 231
    and serotonin, 126
ConsumerLab.com, 181
Correa, Denise D., 67, 69, 71
Cortisol, 100, 158, 205
CT scans, 25–26, 110, 228–229, 230, 233
Cyclophosphamide, 35
    and blood-brain barrier, 94
    and breast cancer, 11, 16, 58, 74, 103, 110
Cytarabine, 87, 88
Cytokines, 8, 168, 208, 227–228, 235
Cytotoxic drugs, 16, 17, 233–234

Dalai Lama, 169
Daunorubicin, 189
Davidson, Richard J., 169
Davidson, Peter, xi
Dementia, 21–22, 113–114, 166, 177, 188, 189–190, 215, 234, 235
Depression
  and acupuncture, 166
  and anxiety, 128
  and beta-carotene, 185
  and bipolar disorder, 11
  and brain, 24, 121, 124–129
  and caffeine, 147
  and cancer diagnosis, 8, 121
  and chemotherapy, 21, 24, 36–37, 55, 58–59, 63, 75, 100
  and chemotherapy: and hormones and menopause, 101, 102
  clinical, 58–59, 122
  and cognitive impairment, 58–59, 63, 64, 121–123, 156, 205
  and cognitive therapy, 123–124
  drugs for treating, 100, 123, 124–130, 131, 140 (see also Mood elevators (dietary))
  and fatigue, 55, 57, 59, 128
  and hospitals, 219
  and imbalances, 122
  and insomnia, 134–135
  and meditation, 170
  and omega-3 fatty acids, 178
  and physical activity, 216
  and "sick syndrome," 228
  and yoga, 167, 168
Dexamethasone, 16, 40
Dexmethylphenidate hydrochloride, 151, 153, 154, 155, 216
Discoveries (magazine), xv
Docetaxel, 110
Docosahexanoic acid (DHA), 174–176, 177–178, 179, 181, 208, 210, 211, 223

Doctors, drugs, and hospitals (avoiding), 218–220, 222, 223
Dopamine, 125, 126, 127, 129, 132, 208, 216
Doxorubicin, 26, 35, 231
  and breast cancer, 16, 23, 58, 74, 103, 110
  and coenzyme Q10, 189
Dysthymia, 130, 147

Egasti, Lois, 4–5
Eicosanoids, 181
Eicosapentaenoic acid (EPA), 174–176, 178, 179, 181, 208, 210, 211, 223
Einstein, Albert, 81–82
Endocrine therapy, 64, 73
Endometrial cancer, 32, 113
Endorphins, 165
Environmental Protection Agency, 179
Epinephrine, 126, 157
Epirubicin, 16
Estradiol, 117
Estrogen, 100, 117
  and brain, 98, 103, 111, 114, 115, 116
  and chemotherapy, 10, 17, 101–102, 103–104, 111
  and cognitive function, 101–108, 111–112, 114, 116, 117
  and ginseng, 149
  and heart disease and strokes, 113, 114
  and hot flashes, 112
  and puberty, 101
  and tamoxifen and other hormonal therapies, 12, 17, 18, 89, 106–108, 110, 113, 114
Etoposide, 16, 40
European Prospective Investigation into Cancer and Nutrition (EPIC), 213–214
Executive functioning, 44–46, 53, 62, 67–70, 84, 97, 103

and brain, 45, 46, 84, 97, 103
and measuring problems, 62, 67–68, 69, 70
Exemestane, 17
Exercise, 139, 163, 164–166, 183, 191, 195, 202, 203, 215, 217, 236, 244

Farris, Donna, 160, 162, 163, 245
Fatigue, 162
  and chemotherapy, 4, 21, 55–58, 75, 92, 101
  and cognitive problems, 8, 55, 56, 57, 63, 138, 143, 144
  and cytokines, 168, 228
  and depression, 55, 57, 59, 122, 128
  and dopamine, 125
  and exercise, 165
  and hormonal therapy, 117
  incidence of, 143
  and nonprescription remedies, 144–150
  and prescription drugs, 150–155
  and yoga, 167
Fats
  and daily limits, 208, 209, 223
  omega-3 and omega-6 fatty acids, 174–183, 188, 190, 208, 210, 211, 222, 223
  saturated and trans, 172–174, 183, 208, 223
Fear
  and cancer, 59–60, 156, 161, 162–163, 167
  and cognitive problems, 156
  combating, 160, 161, 162–164, 170, 205
  and depression, 156
Ferguson, Robert J., 38, 48, 57, 194, 244, 247
Fish oil supplements, 178, 179, 181
5-fluorouracil (CMF), 11, 16, 58, 87–88, 94
Fleming, Peggy, xii

Fluorodeoxyglucose (FDG), 92, 93
Fogginess, viii, xvii, 7, 8, 33, 88
Food and Drug Administration (FDA)
  and Alzheimer's, 100, 127
  and bupropion, 129
  and fats, 173, 208
  and Herceptin, x–xi
  and modafinil, 151, 152, 234
  and Prozac, 128
  and supplements, 179, 204
Ford, Betty, xi–xii
Forgetfulness. See Memory
Foster, Nova, x
Free radicals, 183–184, 185, 186, 188
Fried, Terri R., 23

Gamma Aminobutyric Acid (GABA), 127, 208
Genes, 204–205
Gilbert, Maureen, 56
Gilda's Club, 6, 157
Ginkgo biloba, 189–190
Ginseng, 148–150
Glutamate, 127, 208
Goldberger, Sara, 6
Goldman, Sherry, 5–6, 20, 164
Grape juice, 212, 223
Gratitude, 218
Gum chewing, 196

Hair loss, xv, 4, 95, 233
Hampson, Elizabeth, 104, 116
Hanks, Tom, 105
Healing Odyssey, 160, 161
HER-2, x–xi, 102
Herceptin, x–xi, xv, 231
Holick, Michael, 187
Hormonal therapy, 152, 213
  analysis in Lancet on, 18
  androgen deprivation, 117
  and cognitive function, 8, 10, 17, 75, 114, 117

hormone replacement therapy
(HRT), 112–115
and hot flashes, 112
and sex hormones, 101
and survival, 18
Hormones
and chemotherapy, 98, 101–103
and cognitive function, 98, 101–
112, 114, 116, 117, 122
defined, 99–100
and hot flashes, 112
and prostate cancer, 116–117
and protein, 208, 209
and serotonin, 126
sex, 85, 101, 104, 213
stress, 100, 158, 205
two major classes of, 100
See also Hormonal therapy; particular hormones and classes of
hormones
Hospitals, 219
Humor and laughter, 7, 191, 196–197,
218
Hunsicker, Jackson, 47, 95, 226
Hurria, Arti, 72
Hurricane Voices, 4–5, 31, 32, 33, 39
Hussein, King, xii

Immunotherapy, 56
Impulse control, 45, 83
Inagaki, Masatoshi, 88, 91
Information processing speed, 10, 39,
46, 55, 57, 72
and measuring problems, 67, 68
Information retrieval, 46
Insomnia
and antidepressants, 128, 130
and BZs, 130, 131, 140
and cognitive function, 135
and depression, stress, and anxiety,
134–135
and fatigue, 57
incidence of, 134

and menopause, 111
strategies to combat, 139–142
why we sleep, 135–136
and yoga, 168
See also Sleep
Insulin, 8, 100, 208

James, William, 218
Jenkins, Valerie, 73
Journal of the American Medical Associ-
ation, 190

Kaplan, Stephen, 145
Kimura, Doreen, 104, 116
Kohli, Sadna, 151, 152

The Lancet, 18, 81, 228
Language
and brain, 47, 83, 86, 89, 92
and chemotherapy, 16, 47–49, 67,
86
and memory, 52
LaRue, Stefanie, 108–111
Lazar, Sara, 170
Learning
and anastrozole, 108
and attention, 49, 50
and brain, 103, 105, 116, 126, 127,
164
and chemotherapy, 10, 34, 91
and chemotherapy: and hormones
and menopause, 102, 103
and chemotherapy: studies, 72, 74,
88
and memory, 50, 62
and modafinil, 151
and omega-3 fatty acids, 177, 190
and reversing deficits, 235, 236
and sleep, 136–137
Letrozole, 17, 110
Leukemia, 22, 32
Leuprolide acetate depot (LAD), 106,
107

The Longevity Bible: 8 Essential Strate-gies for Keeping Your Mind Sharp and Your Body Young (Small), 195
Loss of self, 32–33, 34
Love, Susan, 5
Lung cancer, 22, 32, 116, 230
Lycopene, 184, 185
Lymphedema, 167
Lymphoma, 22, 32, 35, 167, 168, 230

MacLean, Paul D., 79
Maki, Pauline, 105–106, 111–112, 113, 114, 117
MD Anderson Cancer Center, 63, 71, 168
Meditation, xiv, 167, 168–171, 195, 206, 250, 253
Melanoma, 22, 49, 230
Melatonin, 132, 141
Memorial Sloan-Kettering Cancer Center, 6, 21, 67
Memory
  and androgen deprivation, 117
  and attention, 49, 50, 51, 62, 69
  and beta-carotene, 185
  and brain (see Brain: and memory)
  and BZs, 131
  and chemotherapy, xv–xvi, 4, 6, 7, 11–12, 15, 20, 36, 39, 40, 41–42, 44
  and chemotherapy: and fatigue and depression, 55
  and chemotherapy: and hormones and menopause, 98, 102, 103, 107, 110–111
  and chemotherapy: and types of memory, 50–53
  and chemotherapy: measuring problems, 61–70
  and chemotherapy: monitoring during treatment, 25
  and chemotherapy: recovering, 235–237
  and chemotherapy: research on, 9–10, 16, 21, 33, 48, 72, 73, 74, 75, 88, 89–90, 226, 228
  computer games for, 195
  declarative and procedural, 50–52
  and depression, 121, 122, 123
  encoding, 52, 53, 68, 69
  and estrogen, 98, 102, 103, 105, 106, 108, 111, 112, 114, 117
  and ginkgo biloba, 189–190
  and gum chewing, 196
  and LAD, 106
  and learning, 50
  and modafinil, 98, 151, 152
  and oral chemotherapy drugs, 22
  and other factors, 8, 11
  and scans, 231
  short-term (working) and long-term, 53
  and sleep, 136, 137
  and stem-cell transplant, 6
  and tamoxifen, 107, 108
  training, 48, 195
  and Vitamin B12, 188
Memory and Attention Adaptation Training (MAAT), 48, 195
Menopause, 19, 75
  and chemotherapy, 10, 98, 99, 101–102, 103, 111, 117
  and cognitive function, 98, 102, 106, 114
  and sleep, flashes, and sweats, 57, 98, 102, 111–112, 134
  and tamoxifen and other hormonal therapies, 18, 107, 112–115
Mercury, 179, 180, 181
Methotrexate, 11, 16, 17, 58, 88
Methylphenidate, 150–151, 153, 216
Meyers, Christina A., 62–63, 66–67, 71
Milk, 211, 223
Milton, John, 217
Mitoxantrone, 16

Modafinil, 98, 151–153, 154, 155, 216, 234
Monoamine oxidase inhibitors (MAOIs), 130
Mood elevators (dietary), 131–133
MRIs, ix, 88, 91, 105, 110, 166, 169, 196, 228–229, 230
Multiple Gated Acquisition scans, 26, 231
Multiple myeloma, 54
Multitasking, 20, 25, 34, 40, 46, 67, 103, 110, 191
Multivitamins, 186, 188, 207, 210, 223

National Cancer Institute, 134
National Comprehensive Cancer Network, 56
National Institutes of Health, 138
Nature (journal), 236
Nausea, xvi, 4, 57, 166, 233
New England Journal of Medicine, x
Noble, Mark D., 87–88
Noor, Queen, xii
Norepinephrine, 125, 126, 128, 129, 132, 157, 208
Norepinephrine-dopamine reuptake inhibitors, 129
Nurses' Health Study, 141

Oathout, Brenda, 152–153
Omega fatty acids. See Fats: omega-3 and omega-6 fatty acids
Oncologists
    and chemotherapy's effects on brain and cognitive function, xvi, xvii, 4–7, 9–12, 19, 32, 90
    questions to ask them about chemotherapy, 13–27
Organization, 33, 34, 39, 80, 83
Oursler, Charles Fulton, 205
Ovarian cancer, xiv, xv, 32, 59, 187, 230

P25, 235–236
Paclitaxel, 94
PCBs, 179, 181
Peptides, 100, 208
PET scans, 22, 24, 25–27, 89, 91, 92–93, 94, 97, 105, 114, 229–231, 233, 234
Phenylalanine, 132
Phenylethylamine, 186, 209
Phytochemicals, 186
Placebo effect, 64, 204
Post-traumatic stress disorder (PTSD), 3
Prednisone, 16, 35
Preventive health care, 220, 222, 223, 237
Progesterone, 100, 102, 103, 104, 106, 113
Progestin, 113, 114
Prostate cancer, 167, 187
    and age, 22, 116
    and hormones, 10, 112, 116–117
Protein, 207–210, 211, 222, 223, 229

Radiation
    and breast cancer, x, xii–xiv, 11, 74, 110, 144, 145, 152
    and chemotherapy, 15
    and cognitive problems, 64, 74
    and fatigue, 56
    and PET scans, 26, 93, 230
Radner, Gilda, 6
Raloxifen, 105
Randomized clinical trial (RCT), 115, 213
Rasgon, Natalie, 114
Raymon, Nancy, 160, 161–162
Rituximab, 35

Sagan, Carl, 81
Salmon (farmed), 179
Saykin, Andrew J., 21

Schagen, Sanne, 73
Schernhammer, Eva S., 141
Schultz, Malcolm, 170
Selective serotonin reuptake
    inhibitors (SSRIs), 126, 128–129,
    206
Selenium, 184, 185
Serotonin, 125, 126, 127, 128, 129,
    131–132, 208
Serotonin norepinephrine reuptake
    inhibitors (SNRIs), 129, 206
Sexual activity, 216
Sherwin, Barbara, 105–106
Skin cancer, 187
Slamon, Dennis, x
Sleep
    and brain, 136–137, 138, 206–
        207
    and cytokines, 228
    and exercise, 165–166
    and learning, 136–137
    and memory, 136, 137
    and napping, 138–139
    and narcolepsy, 150, 151
    and pills, 140–141, 142
    REM, 137, 138, 139, 140, 166
    stages of, 137–138
    strategies, 139–142
    why we sleep, 135–136
    and yoga, 167, 168
    See also Insomnia; Menopause:
        and sleep, flashes, and sweats
Small, Gary, 195, 254
SPECT imaging, 229
Spiritual mailbox, 161–162
Spitz, Rabbi Elie, 162
Stem cell research, 97
Steroids
    as class of hormones, 100
    and cognitive problems, 8, 16,
        116
    and cytokines, 227
    and fats, 172

and insomnia, 57
and mania, 12
sex hormones, 101, 104
and sleep, 134
See also particular steroids
Stimulants, 130, 150–155, 234
Stress
    and brain, 82, 127, 157–158, 235
    and cancer, 3, 14, 145–146, 156
    and cognitive problems, 6, 49, 61,
        67, 156
    and cortisol, 100
    and depression, 156
    and fight-or-flight response, 157–
        158
    and free radicals, 183
    and ginseng, 148
    hormones, 100, 158
    and insomnia, 134, 135
    and protein, 208
    techniques to combat, 159–171,
        205, 206, 212, 215
Supplements, 186–190, 203–204
    See also particular supplements

Tamoxifen
    and cognitive problems, 11, 12, 17,
        72, 89, 90, 105, 106–108, 110
    and survival and side effects, 18
Testicular cancer, 39
Testosterone, 40, 100, 101, 103
    and male brain, 115–116
    and prostate cancer, 10, 112, 116–
        117
Thyroid problems, 101
Transposition, 33
Trastuzumab, x
Tricyclics, 129
Tryptophan, 131–132
Tsai, Li-Huei, 235–236
Tulandi, Togas, 106
Twain, Mark, 205
Tyrosine, 132

UCLA, xv, 108, 202
  and Alzheimer's, 97, 177
  and breast cancer, x, xi, 5, 17
  and chemotherapy drugs, 94, 233–234
  and cognitive problems, 20, 63, 89, 194
  and depression, 24, 121
  and simple behavior modification, 164
  and yoga, 167
Uterine cancer, 87
The UV Advantage, 187

Vardy, Janette, 32
Venlafaxine, 112
Veteran's Administration, 63
Vinblastine, 16
Vincristine, 16, 35

Vitamin A, 183, 184, 211
Vitamin B, 132, 185
Vitamin B12, 188
Vitamin C, 132, 184, 185–186
Vitamin D, 113, 175, 183, 187–188, 211
Vitamin E, 184, 185

Wefel, Jeffrey S., 9, 71, 72
Wellness Community, 5, 6, 157, 170
Winocur, Gordon, 88
Women's Health Initiative (WHI), 105, 112–113, 114, 213
Wooden, John, 202
Word recall and retrieval, 33, 38, 47–49, 57, 68, 83, 92, 106, 231

Yoga, 167–168, 195, 249, 250
Young Survivors Coalition, 10

14